TRAUMATIC BRAIN INJURY HANDBOOK

TRAUMATIC BRAIN INJURY HANDBOOK

HOW A NEAR-DEATH FALL LED ME TO DISCOVER A NEW CONSCIOUSNESS

JOSEPH B. HEALY

Skyhorse Publishing

CONTENTS

I

"OH, YOU'RE AWAKE"

Scientists refer to the ocean environment as inner space; in this way, exploration of the sea or its depths is inner-space exploration. We all know that outer space is that which is beyond Earth's atmosphere or gravitational pull—it is otherworldly. Both realms invite study and encompass mysteries. In both cases, we are eager to go there.

But what about inside *us*, that which makes us *who we are*? Could that be called—interior space? Space is defined as "boundless or indeterminately finite." So by definition our interior space is the function of our brain. The energy produced by this organ engenders our mind, all of our thoughts and emotions, and impels us to any and all action. Some spark occurs and we think or move. That spark is an exchange of neurotransmitters at a junction between neurons called a synapse. A spark or series of sparks happen when we blink our eyes, or cough, or wave, or say "I love you." When we say those words, something stirs inside us, too, and we feel a shudder through our nervous or limbic system, maybe a tightening of stomach muscles or a fluttering in the stomach. This happens instantaneously and you don't *do* it: you don't will it, the action just occurs. That's emotion. Or, it might be a reaction if a loved one says *I love you* first.

The brain and the mind are intertwined. But stuff happens first in the brain, scientists agree on that, at least for the most part they do.

1

Some chemical is emitted or some energy is created in the network of nerves in the brain matter. We move, react, speak, blink. We snap into being who we are. A neuropsychologist said to me simply, "The brain affects everything." I had truly never thought about that until I was forty-four years old and woke up—my term for regaining conscious-ness—after almost three weeks of nothingness. Nothingness—except some incredibly vivid dreams, mainly of water and water scenes such as fishing. I grew up on a lake, and I love to fish, and have spent much of my career producing fishing magazines. These images were safe and familiar to me, or they are to my brain. These memories reside in my long-term memory bank, stored and awaiting recall when needed. I needed them in the summer of 2012 as I wasn't laying down new memories; my brain wasn't capturing any. Therefore, I have no mem-ory from the afternoon of August 14 to approximately sometime on September 3 of that year.

I remember noticing movement up in a maple tree as I sat at my desk in my home office; nothing unusual, maybe it was a gray squirrel or a bird fluttering. I looked closer and it was a cat—our small black house cat that had snuck out of the house and had been outside for days. It was Tuesday, August 14 (I do remember that) and I had been immersed in work, distracted by reading and reviewing email when I noticed the cat. I couldn't believe it was up in a tree in plain view through the window proximate to my desk; I was sure it had been eaten, a healthy morsel for a coyote or a fox or a fisher cat. I had to do something, and remembered the extension ladder—it may have been already outside. This would only take a minute and my wife—the cat person in our family—would be so relieved that the cat was home and okay. This was the cat my wife had trapped when it was a kitten in a neighbor's barn and she nurtured it into a reluctant house cat, shortly after her previous cat of eighteen years had died. I wanted my wife to thank me and to view me in a heroic way, something of a savior. I remember a deep exhale, a kind of "Oh, shit, I guess I have to . . ." feeling of resignation. What came next? The doctors stopped calling it a coma (though my medical records say I was put into a medically induced coma for a short while) and now refer to it as post-traumatic amnesia. Apparently, I was interacting with doctors and walking and pulling out IV tubes. I was complaining of pain in my right wrist, my medical records tell me; it turns out, I damaged my right wrist, I suppose bracing or protecting my body during the fall. I don't remember falling off the ladder or out of the tree. I don't remember voices asking me if I was okay, or my wife splashing me with water to wake me up. I don't remember being intubated (turns out by our neighbor, who in addition to being a science teacher at the high school at which I worked is also an EMT), or the ambulance ride to the nearest hospital or the helicopter ride to Dartmouth-Hitchcock Medical Center in Hanover, New Hampshire. I remember nothing.

The physicians assessed me as an eight on the Glasgow Coma Scale (GCS) after the fall; later that night, that observation was reduced to a 6T (the T meaning intubated, and with the tube down my throat, I'm sure I looked pretty bad). On the GCS, a dead body is generally a three. You, my reader, are a fifteen.

The Glasgow Coma Scale is the scoring system used to indicate the level of consciousness after a traumatic injury. The test involves factoring eye opening (E), verbal response (V), and motor response (M) so that the E + V + M sum results in the GCS assessment: The lower the number, the worse the medical prognosis. A therapist told me the GCS was used to gauge my recovery, as it's a measure of awareness leading to normalcy. So all along the way in the hospital, as I progressed through my amnesia and afterward, I was somewhere on the scale. When I learned I was a six, I was freaked out—that's three points from dead, right? Not exactly, I learned. It's a diagnostic measure but not a prognosis. It indicates the severity of the incident or accident, but it doesn't measure (and no expertise can) the actual physical damage, and certainly is no indicator of cognitive impact or damage, though the verbal and motor components tell medical personnel at least a little bit.

My wife kept a notebook with her when she visited me in the hospital. I tried to speak on August 18th and told Robin I loved her and gave her a kiss. I also said "no noise." A neurologist showed Robin my charts and the images of my head. Even to her untrained eye, she writes, you could see the large spot on the left lobe of my brain, the area the doctor told her controlled speech function and writing. In those early days following my fall, my wife showed me a picture of my son and I said his name, *Teagan,* or something close to it, she wrote.

I've seen a picture of me from that time, with tubes in my mouth and my hands bandaged (so I wouldn't pull out the intubation tubes). I not only looked in bad shape; I *was* in bad shape. I was a virtual Humpty Dumpty, no doubt, who had had a great fall. It was a tremendous lucky break that I fell on lawn and not on concrete. I was lucky. No, I was blessed, somehow and for some reason. As I sit here, my only explanation is I feel I'm achieving my destiny writing this book. Out of all the possible books I might write in my life—all the novels I have written (none published but the work was done) or have begun to write, all the fly fishing or bird-hunting books, all the poetry with which I've dabbled—this is the book I *have* to write, am obligated to write.

"Oh, you're awake." That's my memory of my first moment gaining awareness at Fanny Allen rehabilitation hospital in Colchester, Vermont. It was Monday, September 3, 2012—twenty days after I went up the ladder in my side yard. It was Labor Day, I learned from a TV broadcaster. I was told I would start therapy the next day. My internal reaction was: Okay, if I have to. I didn't know what therapy would be for.

My right arm was in a cast and looking around this was apparently a hospital, so I knew something bad had happened. There was no nagging sense of doom or guilt, so somehow I knew this situation wasn't caused by some badness I had committed. (My Catholic upbringing fostered lifelong acute internal feeling of guilt.) I don't remember anything further from that day. It was September 3, I was in a hospital, and I would have therapy the following day.

I met with Chelsea in an office the next day at 7:30 a.m., led there by a woman I remember as Ludmilla, the kindly nurse with an Eastern

European accent. One of the first orders of business with Chelsea was to start a memory journal, she called it, in a black-marbled-cover Mead Composition notebook, one hundred sheets and two hundred pages, wide ruled—exactly the notebook I had used for years as a journal for writing ideas, poems, kernels of thoughts, transcriptions from the Upanishads, and other sources of inspirational doggerel, outlines of short-story ideas, or examples of writing I might use for later inspiration or guidance.

My longest-surviving notebook as an adult began in 1992 in New York City. In it, like a good Catholic school boy I wrote my address and phone number on the inside front cover: 633 2nd Avenue, #4, NY NY 10016, (212)725-2885; later to change to 331 West 16th Street, #2 and (212)727-0748. The first entry in that notebook was a poem in syllabic verse (so my note says) written at the Mid-Manhattan Library, my frequent weekend refuge when I felt the compelling urge to begin to work as a writer. Also, it cost nothing to sit in the library, which was as much as my budget at that time allowed. If it was the day after a Friday payday, I would sometimes move to Central Park with a paper-bag-wrapped twenty-five-ounce can of beer (or two).

Being surrounded by books in the library was incredibly reassuring. I began to explore those books and discover literature like Tolstoy, which led me to Chekov, Foucault, Henry James, Proust, J. P. Donleavy, as well as *The Epic of Gilgamesh*, by the study of which I began to frame an idea for a generational novel I soon titled *Earthly Paradise*, after the further quest of St. Brendan or Bréanainn of Clonfert to find the Earthly Paradise, which I also learned about in the Mid-Manhattan Library. During this time, I wrote down a quote by T. S. Eliot: "Time past and time future/What might have been and what has been/Point to one end, which is always present." Writing this now, I learn that it's from "Four Quartets," which I didn't make note of in my New York City journal. (Today, I know this is appreciation of awareness and finding the present compelling, which I've recognized through my meditation practice.)

Having just reacquired my present on September 3, my new memory journal would help me remember daily obligations and thoughts.

The past twenty days of my history were gone, unrecorded in my own mental process and therefore never existed, as far as I knew. The "Now" we wrote (Chelsea did the actual writing, as the cast on my right arm made it difficult to hold a pen) at the top of the first page was Fanny Allen Hospital in Colchester, Vermont; next was that my fall happened on August 14, 2012; and that I was admitted first to Dartmouth-Hitchcock and transferred to Fanny Allen on August 29. She then wrote a legend: OT = Occupational Therapy; PT = Physical Therapy; SLP = Speech Language Pathology. I remember observing this with great interest and, in fact, curiosity. "Fascinating" rings in my ear now; and only now I remember it was Mr. Spock who said that on *Star Trek*. I was very much an observer in this situation. I was curious of the present, watching with interest—again, much like meditating on one's own thoughts and studying your own breath, in and out.

According to the journal, on September 4, I met Chelsea first thing, in a therapy room at 7:30 a.m., and we played Connect 4 and worked on organization and visual-spatial tasks. Next, I worked with Ashley on reading, finding words, and putting stories in order. I must have had lunch—we ate in a patient cafeteria; the food is not memorable, even if I could remember—and then at 2:30 p.m. met with Mary Ellen to work on path-finding in the rehab unit, finding my way to the dining room (yes! I was here a little while ago!), going to the gym, and then back to my room, #2029. I kicked a soccer ball forward and backward—maybe I shouted; then again, I don't think so "I played NCAA Division I soccer in college, people!"—and someone told me I did great on my balance.

All in all, this was a successful first day of rehab. Soon, I started to think about the word: Rehab. Mentally and physically, I needed it. Emotionally, my minor successes at, say, simple arithmetic (of the 4 + 6 =10 variety) filled me with a spirit of motivation.

The next day I had a visit from my wife, Robin, and my son, Teagan. Much later, I learned that Teagan found me at the bottom of the ladder when my wife brought him home from day care. "Daddy," he told me, serious and somber, as four-year-olds can be—"I jumped on your chest. I thought you were sleeping."

I don't remember the hospitals at all, until I "woke up." My wife tells me I always brightened when she and my son arrived. We probably watched TV and then I napped. I was allowed lots of naps; I needed them. I tired quickly, as my brain recovered from the impact of my fall, which I learned was characterized as traumatic brain injury.

I have to mention this also—this type of injury was not foreign to me. While in college in Hartford, Connecticut, I interviewed for and was selected as a cooperative-education student at the public relations department of an advertising/marketing communication agency named O'Neal & Prelle. I had quit the varsity soccer team in 1987 (for a while a dream realized, as University of Hartford competed in NCAA Division I) and maintained my financial aid, allowing me to stay enrolled. But I needed a job. O'Neal & Prelle had agreed to pay me and following my graduation in 1989 they offered me a full-time job as a public-relations account executive. I left the agency when hired at *Outdoor Life* magazine in New York City, a PR rookie going legit into publishing.

But while at O'Neal & Prelle, I had the fulfilling experience of editing *Crossroads*, a glossy twenty-page magazine for New Britain Memorial Hospital in Connecticut. One of the hospital's specialties was providing Head Injury Rehabilitation treating "individuals emerging from a coma or those with higher levels of cognitive functioning." I interviewed patients with traumatic brain injury (TBI) and was humbled by their stories, and fully aware that "there but for the grace of God go I." I understood, even in my invincible early twenties, that this injury could befall anyone—or they could fall or be in an accident, literally, head on—and injure their brain. I learned what concussion was, medically. (I never cared to learn while playing collegiate soccer, why worry? And who cared, anyway, was my feeling at the time. I was invincible, after all.) I also learned what the results of TBI could be. I didn't learn much about the functions of the brain.

It's accurate to say as a journalist I was merely exposed to the concept of TBI.

Now here I was in 2012 in a hospital rehab unit going through cognitive therapy. Literally relearning simple mathematics, even learning what the plus sign (+) designated. It looked familiar the first time I saw + on paper and I immediately knew I was supposed to add the figures but I couldn't conjure the sum; once I could grasp addition, we then did subtraction; and finally multiplication. I wrote in my memory journal "Math Problems" with the figures $3.15 + .45 + .75 = 4.35$. I remember that was difficult, but then again I never liked math. I played Crazy Eights and Connect Four and have a note "reason for games is thinking & problem solving & connecting letters & numbers." Because I had a cast on my right arm, my handwriting in the notebook is barely legible (I don't think that was cognitive impairment—no, I don't think so, anyway) so a therapist, Laura SLP (speech language pathology was her specialty) wrote "We worked on generating specific words and on eliminating words you don't need after you have used them. Excellent focus and I appreciated your diverse vocabulary." That brought me a warm feeling when I read it later. The date was September 8, 2012.

Two days later I returned to modern life . . . by being allowed to check email. At 11:30 a.m. with Chelsea in the lunchroom we used the ward PC to check my Hotmail account. With effort, I remembered my screen name but Chelsea had to set a new password for me. It was September 10—twenty-seven days following my accident, the longest I had gone without checking email since the 1990s. I missed a couple of days during a vacation with my wife to Costa Rica in 2007, but now I had an iPhone and constantly checked email, which was the primary mode of communication at the boarding-and-day high school where I worked. Twenty-seven days without email is incredible to me now, knowing how tied I was to my iPhone and email communication during that time. Incredible. I wonder if I had my iPhone with me on the ladder before I fell? I really don't know. I could have been looking at my phone and email when I missed a step on the ladder or attempted to step onto a tree branch. I have no idea because I have no memory of that day or the weeks that followed. I asked my wife about this and she said she used my iPhone later that night to make calls (one to my boss at the school to report what happened to me) but she doesn't remember how she came to have my iPhone. It was just there when she needed it.

Do I remember anything from that time, any snatches of words or sonic echoes or dreamlike shadows or of being drawn toward the light, as some near-death stories have in common? I do.

I remember water. I remember feeling safe and I remember hearing the voices of my parents and brother and sister, familiar voices heard in an unfamiliar place: The timbre of their voices were familiar sounds. I remember thinking we were at a rented house (it was unfamiliar and foreign, but safe) on a lakeshore. It was a lake because I smelled the musty odor of water or moisture. I grew up on a lake, so that was a familiar odor every night of my childhood. I remember seeing the placid surface of a flat-calm lake. I remember being in the Adirondacks, for some reason it evoked Old Forge, New York, or maybe Schroon Lake or Paradox Lake or Lake George or Cranberry Lake. I knew I had been there before. It was safe. I was going fishing with my friend Harry Bowen, I remember that. I remember watching Harry fly cast while he waded along the shoreline. I was happy and excited to have this safe place all to myself. It felt precious, a gift, exactly how I felt about being in the Adirondacks and northern New York as a child. I have these as vivid memories today.

I think now that these were scenes created by my amygdala to keep me calm. No doubt, some memories of the Adirondacks from my youth were being recycled and replayed to transport me to a safe reality. I was a flight risk, under constant watch at the hospital as I had been pulling the IV tubes out of my arm and trying to flee (to where, who knows? I guess, just away from the hospital situation). Fight or flight: My mind, my brain chose flight.

My recovery continued. I was told I would be released on September 12. I worked on word puzzles, deduction problems, math.

The plan changed, Chelsea told me. First, I would go on a field trip and then I would be leaving the hospital on September 17 or 18. And we would make an apple crisp in the kitchen! That was good practice, the therapeutic thinking went, for daily living.

Now that I was back on email, I couldn't resist sending email to my boss and colleagues and telling them I was okay and would be back soon. I had already missed the start of school and boarding-student orientation and I felt guilty about that, my sense of responsibility pushing or willing me deeper into recovery. I remember slowly and deliberately typing the email to a colleague, asking if she had heard about my accident? Of course she had, she answered later that day. I realized it was Sunday, but that never mattered, there were no boundaries or policies on sending email, it was after all the main mode of communication among staff members.

Time moved slowly over the next week, after I showered (I enjoyed the feeling of success wrapping my cast to keep it dry, every day!) mornings were spent in therapy—Occupational, Speech Language Pathology, Physical—and after lunch and conversation with other patients, very much like sleep-away camp, afternoons were spent napping, writing in my memory journal, watching television, and listening to music, particularly Grateful Dead CDs, which my friend from work David Hale, head of the school's Culinary program in the Career and Technical Education department, gave to my wife. *Skeletons from the Closet* was comforting and I recalled many of the words and would surprise myself with what I remembered. Apparently, my wife told me, when I was semiconscious I would play air guitar and mouth the words to songs and I always responded particularly animatedly to the Grateful Dead playing on a boom box. It must have been the high notes from Jerry and that booming bass by Phil, the swirl of melody and harmony; possibly also the ethereal and gritty themes, familiar to me from decades of intense listening to the Dead, memorizing the tunes and attaching meaning to the memories of hearing the songs from the times and places in which I heard them—in my brother's apartment in Clinton, New York, or on our lawn on the shore of our lake, or in a boat on the lake, or in a tent, or the back of a car at an actual Dead show in Hartford, Buffalo, or Rochester.

I had an immediate reaction to the news about my release date: I passed! That's how I felt, much like Charlie Gordon in *Flowers for Algernon*. "Im gonna try to be smart. Im gonna try awful hard." I don't say that to be funny; rather, I'm agreeing with the themes explored in *Flowers for Algernon,* which I read at a young age . . . and I was aware of having the need to prove my smarts again, to prove myself.

On September 17, my wife picked me up at the hospital, we went to lunch at a chain restaurant, went shopping at a supermarket, and then, after a month and a half, I went home. It felt so good to be home, the wafting smells and the scuff of my socks on the carpeting. It also felt safe. I was alive and now safe at home, a few days more than a month after my fall.

2

TRAUMATIC BRAIN INJURY

The brain is *us*, our essence, who we are. It's a mass of nerve tissue (neurons with interconnected filaments called dendrites and axons and glial cells) and blood vessels and is awash in chemicals and proteins and it extends toward the heavens and blossoms out from the spinal cord. The results of the processes of the brain determine our personality and mental ability, our cognition, our intelligence. The brain at work makes us smart or, failing that, average, or plain unintelligent, which is really an interpersonal measure or judgment of reasoning and intuition. (Stupid seems something else, as when you have intelligence but decide not to apply it; dumb means reticent or nonverbal, or even quiet by choice; and then there's apathetic, another layer altogether.) Your brain can storm in a group, it can drain and leave a societal void, it can become sick and get you committed, or literally get a fever like meningitis and become inflamed by virus or bacteria. It's an amazing, remarkable, incredible, truly miraculous organ.

An adult human brain weighs about three and a half pounds and on average is about two percent of our body's weight. Yet it accounts for all of our performance abilities and efforts and peculiarities and individualities and brilliance. *The brain is our totality.*

Our brains are well protected by the skull, which is about six and a half to seven mm thick. However, our bony armor works against us when we fall or suffer an impact to the head, as the soft brain tissue slams against or bounces off the skull, causing bruising (as with concussions) or contusions or hematomas (severe bruising and bleeding with traumatic injuries) in closed-head cases, both of which affect how the brain operates, either momentarily or over longer terms. A handbook given out by Fletcher Allen health care (now known as The University of Vermont Medical Center, the healthcare network where I was admitted for rehab in 2012 after my fall) says that areas addressed in rehabilitation include "mobility, activities of daily living, communication, cognition (thinking skills), perception, swallowing, health management, emotional adjustment, recreation, and return to work/community."

In medical terms, traumatic brain injury occurs from external causes, as opposed to internal causes such as a tumor. A concussion is a mild TBI, symptomatically. Next in the scale after mild are moderate and severe. The common result of a blow to the head is you see stars or have dizziness, a headache, blurred vision, ringing in the ears, a funny taste in your mouth or feel nauseous, and become tired or lethargic. You may have difficulty remembering or concentrating or holding thoughts; you may seem *fuzzy*. You might have difficulty sleeping, as the brain "percolates" to recover regular function. You may be unsteady, as a blow to the head can affect your semicircular canal and interfere with your ability to balance. Due to all of this, you also may get irritable and cranky: you just don't *feel* right.

A person with a mild TBI may remain conscious or may experience a loss of consciousness for a few seconds or minutes. The National Institute of Neurological Disorders and Stroke tells us:

Anyone with signs of moderate or severe TBI should receive medical attention as soon as possible. Because little can be done to reverse the initial brain damage caused by trauma, medical personnel try to stabilize an individual with TBI and focus on preventing further injury. Primary concerns include insuring proper oxygen supply to the brain and the rest of the body, maintaining adequate blood flow, and controlling blood pressure. Imaging tests help in determining the diagnosis and prognosis of a TBI patient. Patients with mild to moderate injuries may receive skull and neck X-rays to check for bone fractures or spinal instability. For moderate to severe cases, the imaging test is a computed tomography *(CT)* scan. Moderately to severely injured patients receive rehabilitation that involves individually tailored treatment programs in the areas of physical therapy, occupational therapy, speech/language therapy, physiatry (physical medicine), psychology/psychiatry, and social support.

Approximately half of severely head-injured patients will need surgery to remove or repair hematomas (ruptured blood vessels) or contusions (bruised brain tissue). Disabilities resulting from a TBI depend upon the severity of the injury, the location of the injury, and the age and general health of the individual. Some common disabilities include problems with cognition (thinking, memory, and reasoning), sensory processing (sight, hearing, touch, taste, and smell), communication (expression and understanding), and behavior or mental health (depression, anxiety, personality changes, aggression, acting out, and social inappropriateness). More serious head injuries may result in stupor, an unresponsive state, but one in which an individual can be aroused briefly by a strong stimulus, such as sharp pain; coma, a state in which an individual is totally unconscious, unresponsive, unaware, and unarousable; vegetative state, in which an individual is unconscious and unaware of his or her surroundings, but continues to have a sleep-wake cycle and periods of alertness; and a persistent vegetative state (PVS), in which an individual stays in a vegetative state for more than a month.

With more serious head injuries, you might have difficulty with your recent memory. Your mind is okay in that you can remember distant events in your thought continuum (long-term memories); however, the new stuff is more challenging to grasp and impossible to recall. This may be amnesia, an interruption in how you record and store memory. The brain isn't recording what's happening to you, in other words. The jostling of the brain has caused a disconnect in the memory process. Doctors described this to me as the brain "not laying down memory," and I experienced it for weeks. In this state, as far as the patient knows, the recent past never happened and there is no yesterday or tomorrow.

These symptoms of TBI tell the story of your injury and are generally grouped as somatic, cognitive, and emotional-behavioral. EMTs and doctors observe and evaluate patients on the Glasgow Coma Scale (GCS), the system commonly used to rate consciousness following TBI. This gives medical professionals a scale of severity by which to judge a patient, which is largely subjective but nonetheless helpful to medical personnel. On the night of my injury, as I've mentioned, I was an eight on the GCS and then was reevaluated as a 6T, but then again I was intubated (that's the T in my score) so couldn't talk so didn't have any verbal score and probably didn't open my eyes. When I first noticed the term GCS in a medical report about me, I looked it up and saw that three or four was considered dead so I inferred that a 6 was exhibiting near-fatal symptoms. It was serious or critical, no question. Based on the GCS, one of my doctors at Dartmouth-Hitchcock Medical Center told me that, at the time of admission, the lower the number, the higher the expected mortality; the higher the number, the better the patient's chances of recovery. I was medically in bad shape.

More useful or evidentiary for doctors leading into my recovery was knowing the duration of my unconsciousness. As far as my memory goes, I was unconscious for about three weeks. But I know now that I was interacting with hospital personnel and my family during this time: I've seen photos of that and heard lots of stories, even though I don't remember any of it. Medically speaking, the book *Communicating Prognosis (Core Principles of Acute Neurology)* by

Eelco F. M. Wijdicks, Professor of Neurology, Mayo Clinic College of Medicine; and Chair, Division of Critical Care Neurology, Mayo Clinic, Rochester, Minnesota, says that:

> Traumatic brain injury results from a sequence of events and includes rapid changes in the cytoarchitecture of the traumatized neuron. Primary axotomy is the result of the mechanical insult, and secondary axotomy is a phase caused by pathological changes within the axon, resulting in major biochemical changes. The node of Ranvier is the weakest part of the axon, and that is where the disruption is most noticeable, resulting in swelling and eventually cytoskeletal disruption. Axonal transport is quickly impaired, and an inflammatory cascade starts, resulting in secondary neuronal injury.

The book continues: "Any blow to the head may cause an obvious injury, but predicting the degree of recovery is complicated." The text further asks "What are the most relevant clinical, radiological, and physiological factors that determine the likely course of a patient with severe TBI?" By way of a partial answer, Dr. Wijdicks says doctors can look for axonal biomarkers like neurofilament in cerebrospinal fluid or the presence of proteins such as tau or S100B (a marker of glial activation) or glial fibrillary acidic protein (GFAP). Shearing of soft brain tissue often produces the most severe effects, as the forces causing rotational injury (whipping the head around or penetrating the skull) can tear the axons and blood vessels, versus compression or shifting (epidural or subdural hematoma) caused by acceleration or deceleration impact. After the traumatic insult, if contusions occurred, a patient may be at risk for edema, or brain swelling, which will create bigger problems for the brain and can be fatal because the skull cavity doesn't offer much room for brain expansion, and the brain tissue comes under pressure from the skull, leading to disaster.

Databases from head-injury studies called IMPACT and CRASH use information from thousands of patients. International Mission for

Prognosis and Analysis of Clinical Trials (IMPACT), including investigators in Belgium, the Netherlands, the United Kingdom, and the United States, gathered data from more than 40,000 patients. This database includes a Prognostic Calculator that offers predictions for six-month recoveries for TBI patients, should you know the admission characteristics for the patient such as CT Classification, motor score, epidural mass on CT, and several other clinical values. Go to www.tbi-impact.org for more information.

Now a finished clinical trial based in the United Kingdom, CRASH stands for Corticosteroid Randomisation After Significant Head Injury and was "a large simple placebo-controlled trial, among adults with head injury and impaired consciousness, of the effects of a 48-hour infusion of corticosteroids on death and neurological disability" that examined 10,008 randomized patients. Predictors included age, Glasgow Coma Scale rating, pupil reactivity, and the presence of major extracranial injury. Their website says, "Worldwide, millions of people are treated each year for head injury. A substantial proportion die, and many more are permanently disabled." Again, the trial is now over but the database information is available at www.crash.lshtm.ac.uk.

The danger of studying the tabulated results from previous TBI cases too closely, however, is that statistically derived prediction could diminish future patient care levels, as TBI is an individualized injury and no two brains respond to the same types of recovery therapies or even need the same level of medical care and attention.

So a concussion is a mild TBI, but a TBI nonetheless. When I coached soccer for a season at the high school where I worked as the director of marketing (it was a day-and-boarding school, therefore the need for recruitment marketing), we had to take a class in recognizing and diagnosing concussions. Players suffering a concussion (in soccer, usually from head-to-head collisions between players or from the head slamming the ground or possibly the goal, almost never from heading the soccer ball) had to rest from practicing and playing for a game or more. In fact, the qualification for high school coaches to be educated about concussions is required by the Vermont Department of Education; the law states that high school coaches must be aware of:

> [T]he risks of premature participation in athletics after sustaining such an injury, and the importance of evaluation and treatment by qualified health care providers. The law expressly prohibits a coach from allowing a youth athlete to continue participating in a training session or competition associated with a school athletic team if the coach has reason to believe that the athlete has sustained a concussion or other head injury during the training or competition. A coach is not permitted to allow such an athlete to reenter training or competition until he or she has been examined by, and received written permission from, a licensed health care provider to resume such activities.

A report by the Vermont Department of Education cites emergency departments in the United States treating an estimated 173,285 persons nineteen years old or younger for sports- and recreation-related TBI (including concussions); 70 percent of these were youth age ten to nineteen.

The therapists and doctors told me during my recovery that every TBI is individual, because the operator/patient is unique. My brain operated a certain way prior to my fall and they could not predict how my recovery would be or how completely my "normal" function would return or recover. I had never in my life had an IQ test so had no indicative medical functional baseline. The doctors had no report indicating my cognitive functional abilities beyond demographic information (age and occupation, primarily). A neuropsychologist confirmed this to me. They didn't know how "smart" I was prior to my fall. The doctors and care providers used my demographic information, and no doubt experience gained from other patient case histories and my family (mainly my wife), to develop a functional baseline for me. That's how they monitored, tracked, observed, and measured my recovery.

They couldn't diagnose how long my recovery would take, as they could diagnose the bone dislocations in my right wrist that also happened in my fall and the process for healing (which included surgery). I had intracranial hemorrhages (the CT scan plainly showed those) but did not require "neurosurgical intervention" so the doctors didn't have to drain, cut, or probe me or my head or brain, primarily to relieve swelling of the brain. This point fascinates me. A student enrolled at the school at which I used to work fell while skiing, struck his head, and did require surgery to relieve swelling of the brain caused by hemorrhaging. Was I spared a more difficult recovery because no one had to mess with my brain? I think so. I was basically a wait-and-see case, the doctors told me, as TBI cases have to be, since every person's brain functions differently and my neurons and brain tissue would heal differently than the next person. In *Providing Acute Care*, Dr. Eelco Wijdicks of the Mayo Clinic writes that medical professionals have to take quick action in determining the severity of the accident.

> One has to determine early on whether neurosurgical consult is needed and whether an intervention can be anticipated. These are not situations that are 'perhaps' or 'probably.' Urgent neurosurgical indications are often obvious at the time of arrival, usually involving the presence of an acute mass effect and brain tissue displacement. The presence of acute subdural or epidural hematoma is a neurosurgical emergency that often requires evacuation. Any cerebral lesion with mass effect may immediately require decompression. Indications for acute—the same day or night—craniotomy or craniectomy depend on neurologic condition at presentation. Only the presence of pathologic flexion or extension motor responses and absence of several brainstem reflexes as a result of pontomesencephalic damage

may suggest that neurosurgical intervention is not indicated. However in cerebellar lesions these necessarily indicate poor outcome because they may indicate brainstem compression that can be relieved with surgery.

Dr. Wijdicks also writes: "Any comatose patient with a new displacing mass is at high risk of increasing intracranial pressure (ICP) and belongs in an ICU. Most major trauma centers use a fiber-optic intraparenchymal device that measures ICP."

My doctors at Dartmouth-Hitchcock decided I did not need neurosurgical intervention, mainly due to the proximity of Broca's area to my hemorrhage and their awareness of what I did for a living (a writer and editor), so they opted to wait for the blood to reabsorb—which it did during the next day or two. I am so thankful that they made this call. That may have been the most important factor in my ability to achieve early recovery within a relatively short (about six months) period—that the doctors did not have to use an invasive method to relieve pressure inside the skull caused by brain swelling. Decompressive craniectomy is a procedure in which part of the skull is removed to allow ICP relief for the swelling brain and that also improves cerebral perfusion pressure and cerebral blood flow. The bone flap is removed and the brain swells, until the swelling recedes and the hole is closed by reinserting the skull flap with a craniosplasty.

As a culture, we're progressively learning more about the brain and how it functions, but interior space and what goes on inside our heads remains very much a mystery. Perhaps, it's the greatest human mystery, as the brain is the foundational organ for every individual and every interaction, reaction, and thought we have and act upon. As far as human organs go, if I ruptured my testes or had my penis amputated I could no longer procreate, right? What a shame—but so long as I didn't bleed to death, I would go on living and functioning and contributing to (or detracting from) society. Or, if my heart failed, I could be hooked up to devices that would regulate my heartbeat, or I could get a new heart through a transplant. Same for the lungs.

But mess with the brain, and you're royally screwed. All functions, all thoughts, all memories—*everything about you could change.* This could happen in an instant. You could be getting out of a relaxing shower, dulled and groggy from the steam, your mind moved on to a conference call scheduled at work at 8:00 a.m. the next day, and in this state of mental and physical autopilot you do what you've done every day since you were in your teens, you step out of the shower—not even watching where you're stepping—maybe extending your arm for balance. Only this time, your left foot slips on the soap as you lift your right foot to step out. You reach for the shower curtain, which pulls free of the plastic clips under your weight, and you go down, hitting your head on the metal spout or the toilet tank or bowl or the side of the tub. You might get up pissed that you ruined the shower curtain and now your head hurts; or maybe you have a gash on your head and have to deal with the blood. Or, like me, you might wake up a couple of weeks later, not knowing where you are. A nurse might tell you, as in my case, that therapy starts soon. And your reaction might be, as mine was: Whatever, okay. Or you might never wake up and your last living moment could be reaching for that shower curtain. Or you might live, but never be the same again, because your brain won't function the same. Ever. Again. Imagine it: Accelerating into a fall and the head striking an immovable object (porcelain or metal) causing a trauma resulting in an injury from which the brain never recovers. Or if the brain can recover, in the process it develops new pathways for cognitive transmission and function, and now there is a before and after and you're a different person. Scary—a horror show—particularly because it's real.

We can look at fall dynamics and force of impact:

FORCE OF IMPACT (F1)

$F1 = Wa/g = WG$

Fi = force of impact (pounds force)

W = object weight (lbs)

a = rate of deceleration (ft/s2)

g = acceleration due to gravity (32.2 ft/s2)
G = G-force

You can simplify this, if you'd like, to force = mass x acceleration (F = MA).

Plug in example numbers using your weight, distance you might fall, acceleration and deceleration, and gravitational force—but know also that the brain keeps moving inside the skull when the body stops, striking the inside of the skull and sloshing back and forth. This potentially causes further injury to the brain, so the fall is bad but the ripple effect or pinging back and forth has consequences too by further rattling the brain. After my fall of what I estimate to be twenty or twenty-five feet, based on the height provided by the extension ladder—I could've climbed higher in the tree, but I don't know how high I was and never will—I had left parietal and right frontal intraparenchymal hemorrhages, a left intraventricular hemorrhage, and a right subarachnoid hemorrhage, and some of these injuries could have occurred in the aftershock as my brain "pinballed" in my skull. I have to add that because I extended my right arm during my fall, in a reflexive action, I absorbed some of the energy or deflected some force of impact into my arm, which may have saved my life.

The hemorrhages to the left frontal lobe were the most troubling to doctors when they learned my occupation was an editor and writer, because the left is where the speech center is located for a right-handed person (which I am), and particularly the part of the brain known as Broca's area and named after its discoverer, Pierre Paul Broca, which is responsible for language tasks, a doctor at Dartmouth-Hitchcock Medical Center told me. One of my attending physicians when I was admitted to Dartmouth-Hitchcock and during my recovery period (actually during a checkup following my hospitalization discharge in late September 2012) showed me a CT scan of my head from August 14 and the radiology report states I had intraparenchymal hemorrhages with the largest being in the left frontal lobe, measuring approximately 3.2 x 2.8 cm.

"In right-handed people, the part of the brain that produces speech is Broca's area and the part of the brain that understands speech is Wernicke's area. Broca's area is a little bit farther forward and if Broca's area is damaged, people can't produce speech. They can understand it, but they can't produce it. That's very disabling for someone whose world revolves around words. In your case, it was extremely fortunate that the blood was reabsorbed," a doctor at Dartmouth-Hitchcock Medical Center, a leading acute-care hospital in my area, told me. "The blood [seen in the scan] is a marker for how much injury occurred."

Another indicator is the amount of time my memory did not function and therefore the length of time during which I have no memory—almost a month. "Reflecting back on your injury, it was severe. To tell that, we look at the length of time when you weren't making new memories. This is called post-traumatic amnesia. The length of time for that post-traumatic amnesia is sometimes used as a rough estimate for how severe the injury is and how likely symptoms will persist," said Matt Kraybill, PhD, Licensed Psychologist-Doctorate, Clinical Assistant Professor of Psychiatry: UVM College of Medicine, Fletcher Allen (Vermont) Psychological Services. Dr. Kraybill conducted the neuropsychological examination in December 2012 that allowed me to return to work a month later, in January 2013.

A statement from the National Institute of Neurological Disorders and Stroke (NINDS) says the organization "conducts TBI research in its laboratories at the National Institutes of Health (NIH) and also supports TBI research through grants to major medical institutions across the country. This research involves studies in the laboratory and in clinical settings to better understand TBI and the biological mechanisms underlying damage to the brain. This research will allow scientists to develop strategies and interventions to limit the primary and secondary brain damage that occurs within days of a head trauma, and to devise therapies to treat brain injury and improve long-term recovery of function."

Interior-space function, though, is a mystery made up of many variables. There is no known surgery to repair the so-called circuitry (more accurately called "pathways") in and of the brain. But we're learning more. "People's ability to recover from brain injury is sometimes amazing but other times so frustrating," Dr. Perry Ball of Dartmouth-Hitchcock told me. Other doctors said most recovery would occur for me, if it would at all, within two years of the injury. (When I first wrote this in July 2014, almost two years had passed since I went up the ladder. I feel I'm still recovering, cognitively, though I completed medical therapies and was discharged from care in early 2013.)

One cohort is unintentionally helping: Our soldiers returning from Iraq and Afghanistan with a preponderance of TBI, as a result of the concussive blasts of IEDs and other explosions. These are called the "invisible wounds of war" since brain injury isn't readily seen and often the only physical evidence of trauma would be the accompanying external wounds. Soldiers don't have a missing limb or a visible shrapnel wound, or as in the two World Wars, lung and respiratory ailments from poison gas, or exposure to a toxin like Agent Orange in Vietnam that results in stroke, heart disease, neurologic diseases like Parkinson's, or cancer.

A TBI can be caused by shrapnel, of course; but many more injuries are caused by concussive bomb blasts. We must also consider the post-traumatic stress disorder (PTSD) and depression from all the soldiers have seen and experienced. The brain now begins to function differently than prior to deployment. And every case is individual, there is no clear-cut diagnosis or prognosis. Each case is wait-and-see, just like mine was.

The Armed Forces Health Surveillance Center estimates that since 2000, more than 168,000 in the Army have sustained a TBI; the Rand Corporation has put the estimate as high as 360,000 for US troops through January 2009. Close to 20 percent of all returning troops have PTSD or depression (mental-heath issues) or TBI,

Rand estimates. More than 1.64 million troops have served in the Middle East since September 11, 2001, according to a document by the Rand Center for Military Health Policy Research.

TBI resulting from concussive blasts are much like those caused by falls; they are known as shock-wave injuries. However, penetrating or external injuries are much different. In *Handling Difficult Situations*, Dr. Wijdicks of the Mayo Clinic writes on this subject:

> Management of penetrating injury is far more complicated, in particular when the injury traversed both hemispheres and when the diencephalic structures and mesencephalon are destroyed.

Regardless of the cause of TBI, a critical question for family members of the TBI patient: Will the medical insurance cover rehabilitation? A brain-injured patient needs recovery time and exposure to cognitive therapies, typically only available within a rehabilitation-hospital's curriculum. Needless to say, like most areas of health care, this is not inexpensive, which puts some socioeconomic factors into play. Does the patient have sufficient insurance coverage? The initial emergency care is expensive enough, but the rehabilitation care is longer term and often requires insurance pre-approval, as mine did.

3

THE WAY BACK

"The sign the miles ways to go
here to there and then get home
another way through the hills
a road that no one knows"
—Wyn Cooper, from "The Way Back"

I was home in Northern Vermont in September 2012 and could not
return to work until cleared by my doctors. As I understood the process, the human-resources department of my employer required this
clearance, as I was on disability from work as provided by my insurance carrier, which covered a percentage of my salary during this
recovery time until the doctors okayed my return to work.

This was my goal: returning to work, as soon as possible—though I
must admit I quickly realized that for once in my adult life I had been
given a pass, so to speak: I could sleep, laze, lull, read, vegetate, chill. I was
allowed time away from professional (and most other) commitments
and I realized, quite suddenly, this was a gift as time was the precious
factor I knew I would need in the coming months and maybe years—I
knew recovery wouldn't come quickly and I was ready to work for it.
I had worked full-time since 1989, days after I graduated college, and
apart from one-week vacations and one-week gaps between old jobs
and new ones, I'd never had a break in commitments or professional
responsibilities, much less a pass to work on myself.

I'd also never thought about what an important benefit disability insurance could be. Of course, I was invincible—or so I thought. I was in my early forties, intelligent, driven, successful, and if I ever fell from a great height I would surely bounce back, no problem. The truth is, I never thought about falling from anywhere. However, I did think about the frailties of mankind and had already begun to sketch out a character for a novel who wore a helmet and a jockstrap and protective cup, as his driving fears in life were an inconvenient head injury or a peeving shot to the balls. I thought this was hilarious—a drug dealer and counterfeiter fearing not gangland retribution but a random act of urban pedestrian violence being his greater fear; then again, why didn't we protect our most vital organs? The character lived in New York City in which pedestrian traffic was a constant threat and danger to the unarmored, or so went my budding literary sketch.

Still, this was mid-September, nearing the end of the first full month of work/school and as I sat at home I was occupied with imaginings of all I was missing professionally. I was driven to prove my sound health and that my language and literary abilities were intact (as I was a professional communicator), yet I was also aware something was amiss. I had difficulty finding words, which seemed elusive or at times evasive. I knew *I knew* the word for which I searched yet I struggled to find it and clamp down on it and spit it out; it hovered just beyond the outer edge of my thoughts. The idiom is "on the tip of your tongue."

I became quieter and not so quick with opinions or conversation. My wife said I seemed unemotional during this period; that was assuredly an evasive technique and protective dodge and vain act on my part because I was feeling strong emotions but could not find the words to express them. I wanted to say so much—most of all, I wanted to apologize to my wife—but I literally couldn't. Evidently, I didn't completely escape injury to Broca's area. I had a form of aphasia, a speechlessness or impairment of speech suffered often by stroke patients—or survivors of severe TBIs. This condition is also called Broca's aphasia. It's a deficiency of expression which is exactly what

I did not want to acknowledge and rather desperately did not want to accept. I was forty-four years old, how could I now be deficient, particularly in language, the very skill I made into a career? I was a writer and an editor, and now a public-relations spokesman—a phrase and identity I avoided and shunned but my name was often labeled with the appellation "spokesman" in the local newspaper when they needed attribution in a story about the school, often resulting from a press release I had sent them.

The application of that label became common during weeks of intense and far-reaching media exposure and attention following the murder of a young science teacher colleague at the school. Melissa Jenkins, thirty-three, had received a distress phone call on a Sunday night in March 2012 from the man who used to plow snow from her driveway. The man's car would not start and he wasn't far from Jenkins's house and he and his wife needed a ride, the plea went. It was a trap. They were out to "get a girl," the man later told Vermont State Police. They followed through with this plan and the charges were that they beat and ultimately strangled Jenkins while her two-year-old son slept in a child's seat in her idling car parked nearby. They dumped her body in the Connecticut River (the boundary between northern New Hampshire and Vermont). The man was arrested and confessed to state police. After a long trial—agonizing for local people who knew Melissa, her family, and the couple on trial—the verdict in 2014 was guilty and both murderers are serving life in prison.

I think often of seeing Melissa Jenkins furtively check her profile in the reflection of the glass foyer of the school's music and arts center as I walked behind her onto campus one morning, about a month before she was murdered. She was pretty, she looked attractive, how I wish I would've told her that. After her death, I found pictures on my cell phone of her science class conducting a demonstration of gravity by dropping eggs wrapped in padding from a pedestrian bridge on campus. As the school's PR guy, I shot photos of teachers and students all the time, and never imagined the personal significance of these digital images. (Unfortunately, lost now with that old iPhone.)

While the legal process inched forward and the media attention on the murder exploded, I felt one of my professional responsibilities as the school's marketing-and-communications director in the wake of this horrific crime was knowing the extent to which the school was mentioned or covered in the media. The results were astounding, many millions of media "hits" in the *lingua franca* of media-exposure studies. I enlisted a media monitoring service to tell us exactly where these hits happened and the accrued exposure numbers. The story became international news in a very real version of a media feeding frenzy.

I was the media spokesman whose name was on press releases and media alerts and updates, but the true spokesman during this awful ordeal was the school's headmaster, Tom Lovett, whose wise and calming counsel through the early hours of the teacher's reported disappearance and the discovery of her body and then the arrests of the suspects, kept everyone together. His bonding agent was simple: Love. He expressed love for the students, the faculty and employees, parents, townspeople, alumni of the school—for the larger world. His phrase was Love Wins, powerful and effective and conveying elemental human emotion and empathy. The phrase is hopeful, compassionate, uplifting, and beautiful. Disyllabic and declarative, the phrase became a rallying cry for good at the school and in the Northern Vermont town in which this horrific murder happened.

Melissa Jenkins was murdered at the end of March 2012, leaving all at the school gasping for air and grasping for humanity, and saved by love. As the marketing-and-communications director for the school, I faced relentless queries for information on the case and probing journalistic interest into the school and the town, all the while still maintaining some focus, albeit distracted, on regular marketing matters, like recruiting new high school boarding students from across the world to apply for enrollment. (The school already had boarding students from nearly thirty countries.)

I was numbed by the experience, and being proximate to kids every day made the situation even more surreal for me. I had only a year's experience working at a secondary school and embarked on this job because I thought working with teenage students, teaching them when asked what I had learned in more than two decades in business and journalism, would be rewarding. (I was not a teacher, but I was asked to discuss marketing and media communications in classes, from time to time.) My parents had retired from careers as schoolteachers, Dad at a high school and Mom in elementary school. I thought for sure this would be a fit for me, in my DNA. I never dreamed of this type of tragedy happening—a cold-blooded murder with the woman's two-year-old son sleeping just feet away, the murderers apprehended a couple of miles from my family's house (where our four-year-old son slept), the woman's body dumped and recovered, also a couple of miles from my house, in the icy Connecticut River. We all coped the best we could. Certainly, it brought the staff, teachers, and students closer, as tragedy often can.

Shortly after "matriculating" as marketing-and-communications director at the school, I met with Headmaster Lovett one day and he told me he thought it was time to write a blog on the school's website. I disagreed. I told him point blank: he should write a column that would resemble or actually be based on an address he delivered nearly daily at the school's morning chapel, the nondenominational all-school gathering or assembly with which every regular day started, held in historic Fuller Hall, a theater with enough seating for grades ten to twelve and most of the faculty. This would be the top administrator's view of important or rallying or interesting topics influencing and affecting the school and its students. It was called "Headmaster's Weekly Message: Our Academy" and appeared (as it still does last time I looked) on the school's website home page. It was an important means of communication with constituents interested in the school's affairs, from the head man. At this time of tragedy, Mr. Lovett wrote a column entitled "A New Normal." This appreciation for a new normal was a perspective I adopted later in 2012 after my injury.

We will grieve for a long time. Grieving is a process and not a linear one. It is normal and expected. Some of the stages of grief are:

1. Shock (we can't even comprehend such a thing has happened);
2. Disorganization (we have a huge emptiness in our lives and need to fill it or organize our lives around it);
3. Volatile emotions (these can include sadness, fear, and anger; sometimes we will be in conversations or involved in activities and be suddenly and unexpectedly overwhelmed with strong—even violent—emotion);
4. Guilt (we think about how we could have stopped such a horrible thing from happening or how we could have loved her better or done more for her);
5. Loneliness (we will feel like no one understands what we feel or we will miss Melissa intensely—needing exactly what she brought to our lives—and find there is no one to take her place);
6. Depression (both individually and communally, we will feel a letdown not only from the frenetic pace of last week but from the loss of joy and innocence that Melissa's death has caused; the world will just seem darker and life less purposeful);
7. Reorganization (we will find a way to accommodate this pain like a tree growing with a spike driven through it; the spike is just as big and real, but the tree keeps growing. Some call this "moving on," but it certainly doesn't mean forgetting or leaving Melissa's memory behind).

We will have bad days and better days. Members of our community will grieve differently, for we are a diverse and complex community. As we have shown throughout the past tragic days, we are an accepting, understanding, empathetic,

and loving community. We will come to rely on that goodness daily.

Another part of the "new normal" is that our school has had
a spotlight on us and will continue to be watched. Part of that
will be simply people's interest in how a school copes with such
a loss; but a large part of that interest comes from the fact that
our community has inspired others.

The words we have spoken, the words that we use to honor
and remember Melissa, have resounded around the world—
"love wins," "love those the most who need it the most," "what
lies behind us and what lies before us are tiny matters compared
to what lies within us—and let that be love."

I have received hundreds of emails, phone calls, and notes
from around the world, especially this broken corner of the
world; I have received comments from those who have been
here—including members of the national media—who are
inspired by our love for one another.

Moving forward, I hope—I believe—that this love will
become part of our "new normal" and more people will look at
us and say, "See how they love one another."

I want to offer you some suggestions on how to handle this
new normality—this sense of loss, grief, and love:

1. Get outside and get outside of yourself. Exercise, pray,
   appreciate and look for the goodness around you.
2. Focus on what needs to be done. Serve those who need
   you, do the tasks assigned to you, stay busy with things
   you like to do.
3. Give yourself a break. We will make mistakes, we will
   have bad days, and we will not be able to do all the things
   we used to do. We will be tired and emotional. Don't take
   on too much. Feel free to say no.
4. Give others a break. Forgive mistakes and emotional out-
   bursts. Be kind. Understand that some don't want hugs or

attention and that's OK. Try to understand before complaining or criticizing.

5. Make it to Spring Break. Pull each other along by finding
   fun things to share or things to look forward to. Set short-
   term goals. We have two weeks left.

Finally, part of this "new normal" for me is a new sense of gratitude. I have told you already that last week I fell in love with you
all over again. Today I want to tell you that I am so grateful for
the opportunity to be here with you—specifically and particularly
with you.

We have been here in fun times and sad times and good times
and evil times. But we have been here together. We could have
been here with some one else, but we have been here together.
Out of all the people ever created, we ended up here at the same
time to share these times together. And I have never been more
thankful for anything in my entire life than to have been here
with Melissa Jenkins and to be here with people who knew and
loved her—who were known and loved by her—to be here
with you now, to have the chance to know and love you.

For those who share any of these sentiments with me and
who, like me, continue to grieve, I offer one last thought: I have
sworn to live my life in such a way that I will see Melissa again.
If you do not share the same faith or beliefs that I do, I ask you
to live your life in a way that would make her proud, in a way
that honors her, in a way that makes her life perpetually more
powerful and more meaningful.

I know now I should have sought grief counseling, which the school
made available. Instead, I decided to stay numb. Alcohol was the helpful substance. I tried to keep that at a moderate, numbing intake, but
excesses flared on weekends and after hours. That continued into July
when I got a call from my mother, who once again needed knee surgery,
the prosthesis in her knee giving way yet again. (Both of the joints of her

knees had been replaced several times, going back to my childhood.) My father, who has Alzheimer's and possible cognitive damage from a stroke, couldn't take care of my mother so I flew to Florida to help with her hospitalization and to care for Dad. By August, I was exhausted and had no break from stress for many months. I still sought relief through numbness. By the afternoon of August 14, I had inserted in myself a couple of drinks, I remember that. As any amount of alcohol changes the function of the human brain, I was impaired. I remember seeing the black cat up in a maple tree; I could see that as I sat in my desk chair in my basement office space. I remember thinking, I have to get her down. It was the former feral kitten my wife trapped with a Havahart live animal trap. Robin nurtured it into a house cat; it lived inside the house, furtive, hiding and sleeping most of the day. Occasionally in the summer it would escape outside and it clearly had the instinct to take care of itself. (Though it never grew much larger than a kitten, so it appeared to me to be a helpless kitty lost outdoors as I watched it on that August day.) It had been outside for a couple of days and my wife was beyond worrying, reaching the point of trying to forget about the cat, saying "there's nothing we can do now." *Au contraire!* I could get it down from the tree and bring it back home! From my desk chair, I could see the cat perched on a maple-tree limb. I could get it, I figured, in about five minutes, tops. The biggest pain would be hauling the fiberglass extension ladder down to the tree and setting it up, alone. What if it fell on me, it was solid fiberglass, that sucker would really hurt! Anyway, I dragged it down the lawn. I have a hazy memory of setting up the ladder. My next memory is waking up in a bed in the hospital and being told, "You're awake—good. Therapy will be starting soon." Okay, whatever. I had a childlike acceptance of much that transpired in the weeks that followed.

When I went up that tree, I was a sour, bitter person, generally unhappy about my station in life, definitely dissatisfied. (How absurd to be that way, I can only say now—truly insane.) This was a sourness not directed at anyone but myself, honestly. I was satisfied and happy I had moved my family back to Northern Vermont from the coast of Maine, which never felt like home, and for having a dependable job at the reputable and historic institution of higher learning in an area still known for its menial labor in logging or over-the-road trucking or farming, a job that allowed me to qualify for a mortgage on a well-built house with views of the White Mountains of New Hampshire, including the ski trails of Cannon Mountain. With the right sun we could see the glint off the glass of the gondola house at the top of Cannon. I made this happen, though I harbored an unspoken bitterness that I had given up a pretty good career in magazine publishing to be the PR guy for, I felt at that time, a high school. Not even a college! I justified that decision as being necessary so my family could move back to Vermont and anyway my son would go to this excellent boarding-and-day high school one day, and I knew that my own sense of achievement in a career no longer mattered now that we had a four-year-old child.

Still, I wanted my career to matter, egoist that I was, and I wanted if not to surpass all expectations of secondary-education marketing, then in a hurry to get beyond a nonprofit high school and go into corporate flack-ery, where the real money was.

I look back now and I have to say, simply, I wasn't a good person at that time in my life; by my own definition, I really don't feel I was. I subjugated most of these bad feelings and did what I had to do, but I was not myself, not my true self. I had veered from my core. I was not living right and I knew it but some part of me also didn't care and accepted this negation. Deep down, some part of my being and my consciousness knew I was headed for a life collision.

Having a family to support, money was always a concern and I wanted to earn more because I thought more money would bring more freedom, which had to bring more satisfaction. I loved being a father and I loved my wife (and still do) though I was a prick and overbearing toward her. My son was too young to see any bad in me, and I also loved knowing that and had decided I would change before he got old enough to notice. I had a couple years of being a prick to go, the devil on my shoulder would whisper to me. Or the devil did—until I mounted and climbed that ladder and knocked him the hell off.

The event was a blessing for me, personally. My fall, described by doctors as near fatal, gave me a full appreciation when I woke up of how beautiful and amazing life is and how fortunate I've been. I haven't had hardships. Yes, I've had to work—that was always expected of me by my parents—when I got my working papers at age fourteen. I went to work pulling weeds on a black-dirt potato farm in Canastota, New York, the same as my older brother did before me and my younger sister after me. I never suffered, though I saw my mother suffer with an ulcer and with the knee surgeries she needed after an allergic reaction to ulcer medication degraded the cartilage in her knees. My grandparents died and I lost a couple of close friends to death, when I was in my twenties and thirties. I was reckless as a kid, fell in love with punk rock in high school, and started playing bass guitar to emulate the nihilistic attitude of a punk, though I was raised in a town with one stoplight and a population of maybe a couple thousand people, on a lake, in a rural area of Central New York.

My parents were teachers, and ours was a middle-class family structured around education, striving to be the best. Fully focused on the life of the mind, you might say. I was athletic enough to play Division I soccer in college, I worked in public relations in college (my first experience as a flack, though I was an agency flack so it wasn't the same as being an in-house flack working directly for a company, or in my case an educational institution), and I was hired by a large-circulation magazine in 1992 in Manhattan at a time when a career in journalism was robust if not sexy and pretty straightforward in that it required specialized knowledge (in my case, of hunting, fishing, and outdoors sporting pursuits) and expertise in the language, about twenty years before the word blog was a thing and at that time a web was still something spun by arachnids.

I have been blessed in life and the only explanation I can offer for that is I've been a pretty good person for most of my life. I have no evil intent and though I have my share of pissy and angry moments, those ill emotions are not directed at anyone in a hurtful or spiteful way, and usually would be directed back at me, which I feel has helped me to learn and grow from experience and introspection. I would say I fit neither the profile nor definition of a mean, malicious ass full of ill intent.

I've also had a mind that would never abate or shut off. My entire life, I've had a constant internal monologue, as far back as I can clearly remember, going back to preteens. I always thought intensely about *everything* and would turn those thoughts over and around in my head, nonstop, incessantly. I always wanted to be smarter, better, to know more. I had a facility for learning quickly and I figured this was because my mind was constantly in motion; I couldn't shut it off, and for a long time—decades—I considered it a gift. This made me different from others; it made me an artist.

Later, my interior monologue became a burden and would cause sleepless or fitful nights. And then my hyperactive or obsessive-compulsive mind became an affliction and I could only shut off or manage the incessant thoughts through an intake of booze—the booze cocoon, I called it, cooing as I said it. That behavior became my private fun—private because I knew it was abnormal and, in a Catholic religious sense, wrong. Still, it was strangely fun to manage—to have enough alcohol so my thoughts were lively and entertaining and if I started to realize I had too much alcohol, I learned how to act as if I hadn't. This is what Jack London called "The White Logic," the ignoble sneering at "the phantasmagoria of living":

> "One step removed from the annihilating bliss of Buddha's Nirvana," the White Logic adds. "Oh, well, here's the house. Cheer up and take a drink. We know, we illuminated, you and I, all the folly and the farce."
>
> "Drink," says the White Logic. "The Greeks believed that the gods gave them wine so that they might forget the miserableness of existence."

So my self-created afflictions undeniably included drinking alcohol, at times excessively—which I also thought I could always handle. I freely admit, it provided me succor and relief from constant, badgering thoughts and ruminations. It temporarily would abate and quiet the thoughts and instead help me to focus on a distraction like music or a movie, or enjoyable reading, a break from studying and learning the craft of literature. Alcohol wasn't the sole source of my dysfunction; I had rotten thoughts too. Maybe that was from depression after all? Or simply the accumulated experience of living forty-four years in our modern society?

I began to understand all of this a little bit through weekly sessions with a therapist after my release from the rehabilitation hospital, as a doctor cautioned me that I was at risk for depression when facing life challenges and adaptations—I bristled at the word "accommodations"—in my recovery. More therapy may perhaps tease out more answers about life that begin to satisfy me.

What I know is that when I woke up from my "alcohol-related fall from a ladder," as some the doctors' reports read, I did not crave alcohol. Biologically, my body and my mind no longer craved its effects. Psychologically, I knew I had survived a serious injury and I heeded the doctors' advice when they told me I could not backslide to alcohol use or abuse—the brain could not take it. I truly didn't want to. This wasn't a test of will—will power had no place here—I simply had no interest in feeling drunk, in fact the thought scared me. That was the survivor part of me feeling vigilant. I had a second chance. The sense of being (and the twisted feeling of responsibility to be) an Irishman with a so-called wooden leg was gone. The contributions of the effects of booze to my being a quick and vivid thinker now seem absurd; the booze cocoon was shed, shredded, a discarded chrysalis left behind in the ash heap of time. Incredibly, the craving was completely gone. I imagined this is what a lobotomy must be like, though of course I had no tissue ablation. Maybe this was the result of an injury to the region of Broca's area—the quieting of my internal monologue? It hit me one day during my recovery that something was missing. It was not cognitive function, that seemed to be progressing okay, though my thoughts came to me a little slower. After a morning mindfulness meditation session, it came to me—I was no longer plagued or directed by thoughts from the incessant inner voice. The chatter, the clatter, the nattering had been quiet now for about a year, I realized in autumn 2013.

Following my fall, I was more emotionally expansive. I appreciated (loved and embraced!) life, I understood the power of love though also knew (and still know) that potential evil percolates within our brains and can seep into the powerhouse called our souls (whatever part of the brain that is, though it feels as if it's in our core or center—for example, when we undergo therapy and recover, we talk about being centered).

The craving, I'd say, grew cumulatively over those forty-four years, beginning with my first drink in high school and becoming easier to manage all the time. I came to know the behavioral pathways, but also the cognitive pathways, which led to a craving and need for the effect. In other words, an addiction. "The genial brain glow," Jack London called it in *John Barleycorn*, a book I found tremendously introspective and helpful to me in my recovery. If you've ever thought about having a drink for the hell of it, and of course if you've done it, I recommend you read *John Barleycorn*. If you want to go deeper, read *The Lost Weekend* by Charles Jackson. If you can stomach it, there's always Charles Bukowski—and many other writers of a related genre path from whom to learn both in print and from their actual life.

Today, after my fall, I do not have an internal monologue, it's gone. I can sleep unhampered through the night and feel refreshed in the morning, not nagged by constant thoughts or a cacophony or caterwaul of internal voices. That feels new and is wonderful. Life feels new and is wonderful, every day is truly a gift and I want to contribute the most I can to humanity in the time I have left. I'll turn forty-nine this year. Soon, I'll be fifty and my son will be ten and my wife will be forty-nine. I already mourn a bit for my hunting dog, an English pointer that will be about eleven (he's a rescue dog so we don't know his exact whelping date) when I'm fifty.

The fall was a blessing, it brought me back to my core. I love writing and will write throughout the rest of my days, and with hope I'll continue to do that as well as edit professionally. (I edit a magazine now called *Covey Rise*, about the lifestyle of wingshooting.) I love the act of creation and communicating through words. I could have lost that ability completely, forever. If I had, maybe I could've taken up the bass guitar again and truly learned how to play, this time (unlike when I was lazy at fourteen and was excused from any virtuosity by the three-chord standards of punk rock). I'm lucky in life.

With our magical brains, we have no choice but to consider deities responsible for creating our beautiful brains and senses of touch and smell and life itself. How could it not be so? It could be random evolution, that is true. But it feels beautiful and humbling to consider a higher power guiding and protecting us. Born into the Catholic faith, I had my fill of hearing about the punishment we deserved as fallen human beings, the penury of original sin. Let's live and be happy. Let's love one another. Love truly does win—I learned that, I saw it, I believe it.

In the fall of 2012, I was fascinated and challenged by the process of recovery. As I've said in these pages, I was an eager participant in physical and cognitive recovery. I was out to prove that this injury did not change me—mainly to myself, as no one was questioning me. While at the rehabilitation hospital, I was filled with the drive toward accomplishment much like I felt, myself, in high school about thirty years before. Yes, I worked at a high school so I was in touch with the feeling again each time I walked through the corridors of an academic building or wrote a press release about student achievements or sat in the audience at a play or musical performance, or watched a senior capstone presentation. Certainly, coaching high school soccer the autumn previous to my fall had refreshed that feeling. I had a drive to achieve. At my discharge from the rehab hospital, a therapist mentioned that I had been in an "advance recovery cohort." I was observed and the "teachers" (the doctors!) had judged me an advanced, high-functioning student. I only felt I wanted to do well; I was determined to win back my humanity. There was no adversary as a target for that determination, only a self-awareness that I could improve myself and my own awareness of the value and shared beauty of being alive.

To have this opportunity to get to work rebuilding and remaking myself resulted from the care I received. (A big shout-out to all of the emergency responders and doctors and care providers at the hospitals and offices through which I passed!) Living in one of the smallest-population areas in the second-smallest state by population in the country, I had incredible early medical care, none of which I remember. The doctors joked later and said, "It's better you don't remember, nothing really happened." I think that's the point, Doc. Nothing happened to me, nothing was expected of me, I got a tremendous amount of rest, I had lots of personal attention—peace, rest, care, and emotional support.

Back home, I also was given time—thanks to the disability insurance my employer provided, which I had never imagined I would need. I would not return to my full-time job until the next semester, beginning in January 2013. For the first time in my adult life, I really had no responsibility other than healing my brain and restoring my cognitive function as completely, and as rapidly, as I could. I wanted to put my brain to work and test my functions in daily living and doing the work I loved and felt I was good at—editing language. I seized the opportunity to be an active member of the publishing-advisory team assembled by my friend, the author and photographer Peter Miller, to proofread and give advice on what should run in his excellent, self-published book *A Lifetime of Vermont People.* I had reviewed photographs Peter was considering for the book the day of my accident and appreciated that my help was needed. I line-edited chapters of the book, reviving my love for this process that I had developed while launching the imprint *Fly Rod & Reel Books* for my then-employer Down East Enterprise a couple years earlier.

Due mainly to the sputtering economy leading to our economic recession beginning in 2008 and the accompanying hardships of selling magazine advertising as a publisher in a small vertical market (as fly-fishing is), I had become fatigued with publishing and felt I had nothing more to contribute, and excitedly accepted the offer to join the high school staff as marketing-and-communications director, in 2011. That was after serving as the associate publisher of *Fly Rod & Reel* magazine for three years and watching participation and interest in the sport of fly fishing decline. The career change was welcome, but even more so was the move back to Northern Vermont and the community I had left to move to Maine, which simply did not provide the same sense of community and, though a familiar-feeling New England area, it also never felt like home, not the way Northern Vermont did. I was editor-in-chief of *Vermont Magazine* for five years previously and developed a love for the entire state and its peculiarities and unique place in our fifty states.

When I began to visit Northern Vermont in 2001 to have my hunting dog trained by a professional trainer, I immediately felt a sense of being home, as the area was so much like the Adirondack Mountain towns I remembered visiting with my parents when I was a child. I discovered I could buy a small house on the side of a ski mountain on about an acre of land, for less than $100,000—and I jumped at it. It was the first house I owned, about ten minutes from the nearby winter resort's chairlift, just as I started to get serious about being a snowboarder. I absolutely loved the feeling of floating down a snow-covered mountain, the feeling familiar and meaningful as I had begun waterskiing at a young age. I grew up on a lake in New York State, and this part of Northern Vermont known as the Northeast Kingdom (courtesy of the rhetorical mastery of Vermont Governor and Senator George D. Aiken who reportedly coined that phrase during a public forum in the town of Lyndonville in the late 1940s to give this distant and sparsely populated region an identity) was immediately home. I could not only snowboard minutes from my house; I also could hunt grouse and woodcock walking out my front door. I discovered I had wild brook trout in the small pond on my property and they would take artificial flies, or I could fly fish in the local river or area ponds. I was the editorial director of a group of national fly-fishing magazines that covered freshwater and saltwater fishing, as well as the craft, skill, and art of fly tying. I had traveled a fair amount to fly fish, both in the United States and as far as Mexico, Canada, and Ireland. After a weeklong trip floating the Smith River in Montana in the early 2000s, I vowed to make this sort of life-fulfilling move, though I did feel it would probably be to the Rocky Mountain West.

Here in the Kingdom, a seriously awesome network of single-track mountain-biking trails surrounded my house and Kingdom Trails had included my road as part of the network, so it literally was at the end of my driveway. I was editing fly-fishing magazines when I bought the house, living in southern Vermont, and I began to commute to the Northeast Kingdom about three hours north every weekend. Friends in southern Vermont asked somewhat incredulously, "Why would you move to the end of the road, where the United States runs out?" I would answer, "Exactly."

The next year, 2002, I accepted a job to become editor-in-chief of *Vermont Magazine*, and did that publishing work remotely from the cottage and also from the magazine's office in Middlebury, Vermont. I met my wife while we both were snowboarding on the nearby mountain in the Kingdom. Robin is stunning, matching my height of six foot one, and I found myself paired with her in the singles queue as we waited for the old-time, two-seat chairlift. That was in January 2004. We were married ten months later on Cape Cod, where her family has a vacation house. My wife was working in the Boston area and was accustomed to larger cities, so we took an apartment in Vergennes, Vermont, to be close to my office in Middlebury and also to the one true city of the state, Burlington. She took a job in on-the-road sales and covered Vermont and parts of New Hampshire. I edited *Vermont Magazine* until that reached its end in 2007 and, deciding I couldn't buy out my business partner, I resigned and took a job back in the fly-fishing-publishing business in Camden, Maine, and we relocated there just before my wife gave birth to our son at a hospital in Damariscotta, Maine.

When I was in recovery, healing from a self-inflicted traumatic brain injury, I wondered, *Why did I get to this stage of recklessness?* I asked that of myself every day in the hospital, as I could no longer rely on the involuntary and incessant internal monologue to ask for me. Why was I so careless, imperiling my very life for momentary cognitive relief as I swilled a vodka tonic on a summer's afternoon? On the day I write this chapter, the local newspaper ran the front-page headline "Police: Man In Two-Story Fall Was Drunk And Chasing Pigeons" and the police chief in Littleton, New Hampshire, where it happened, was quoted saying, "The message for this is definitely do not chase pigeons while drunk on a rooftop. It is not a good thing to do for your physical well-being." I would say not, as the man chasing pigeons, thirty-five, wound up being transported to the same hospital I was in 2012. The news report did not list traumatic brain injury as one of the man's many injuries (although collapsed lung and multiple broken bones were).

In the hospital, I worked on mastering the tasks I was given, like simple arithmetic and reading problems and following the rules of Connect Four. I succeeded at these and many more challenges and I was released. I continued to work on cognitive tasks and I rediscovered publishing by helping on a friend's book project, and I wrote a detailed freelance article published in a major outdoor magazine. I continued with math skills and word-finding puzzles, and Lumosity. I played Lumosity with my then four-year-old son and I can't say I was always better or more adept at problem-solving challenges or puzzles. Inside my cerebral cortex, I had more reservoirs of experience stored than my son, and maybe that's what ultimately helped me "to win" in our one-on-one challenges. I did feel a sense as weeks passed that my brain power was ascending.

In early December, after the dislocated bones in my wrist had been surgically repaired and the cast removed, I had the ultimate test: the neuropsychology examination that my attending doctor had required before I'd be allowed to return to work. I spent about four hours with Matt Kraybill, PhD, at the rehabilitation hospital. He put me through the wringer, as he had to by training, to ensure that I was capable of returning to work. We did the Boston Naming Test, the California Verbal Learning Test, the Delis-Kaplan Executive Function System Verbal Fluency, Color-Word Interference, Tower Test subtests, Finger Tapping, Grip Strength, and Grooved Pegboard from the Halstead-Reitan Neuropsychological

Battery; Rey-Osterrieth Complex Figure; Sensory Perception Exam; Wechsler Adult Intelligence Scale and Wechsler Memory Scale Logical Memory subtest (both Fourth Editions); Wisconsin Card Sorting Test-64; Beck Depression Inventory—and many more. It was an exhausting day. I was shaken, truthfully, and didn't know how I did, as I mastered some and floundered through others. I went home and waited. We prepared for Christmas . . . and I received the report—I was cleared.

"Taken together, Mr. Healy demonstrated many good scores across a wide variety of cognitive domains. His overall psychometric intellectual functioning appears to be solidly within the average range and he demonstrated good language functioning, attention, and working memory. However, Mr. Healy had isolated low scores on some measures of processing speed, visual-spatial organization, learning/memory (particularly for nonverbal information) and some measures of executive functioning. Although these patchy low scores do not represent prominent cognitive impairment, they likely represent a decline from his highest estimated premorbid level of functioning (based on his education and occupational achievements as well as his other good scores). This pattern of cognitive functioning is not clearly lateralizing or localizing but is compatible with his history of a traumatic brain injury and bilateral intraparenchymal hemorrhages."

I was cleared! The report concludes: "His specific prognosis is unknown but Mr. Healy may continue to have gradual improvements in some domains of cognitive functioning given that his injury was less than 6 months prior to this evaluation." One recommendation included taking care "to avoid overwhelming himself with too many things or tasks that are very difficult. He should continue to find balance between pushing himself and also being careful to avoid overwhelming himself."

I returned to work at the high school and the staff could not have given me a stronger and more loving welcome back, greeting me with a standing ovation on my first day of the faculty and staff meeting (called "in service") of the semester, 2013. Their welcome and expression of confidence in me was tremendously uplifting. I will never forget it.

On one of my first days back to work, a teacher asked me innocently enough how I was feeling and how my recovery was going. "What percentage would you say you are, compared to before?" he asked, again I assumed earnestly. I wasn't ready for that question. I laughed it off and said something innocuous like, "Oh, it's all okay, the doctors cleared me, that's why I'm back." Then I had a momentary flash of my old self and blurted: "It's a good thing I started at 150 percent, because I guess I'm at 100 percent now!"

The thought dawned on me then: I had needed recovery. In January 2013, I was reconnected to my core, I was myself again. Perhaps my brain was not as "finely tuned" as the moment prior to my climbing the ladder, but I was better now.

What a powerful phrase: I was better now.

The person I was before I climbed that ladder would never have accepted or succumbed to recovery. But I needed to recover, emotionally and cognitively, from some kind of crud that had settled into the folds of my brain.

It was about this time I imagined St. Peter telling God that this Healy guy had to go, that he wasn't contributing anything good to humankind. He had to go. And God (or maybe Jesus—I had been a Catholic altar boy in my teens and served both) had said, No, that wasn't the way. God said, We'll recalibrate this character, set him straight. He pinged me off that ladder and I woke up about three weeks later, remembering nothing about the fall or the ensuing hospitalization, only becoming aware of my need and obligation (to my family, to my wife, to my son) to recover.

Recovery is major, incalculably necessary. It is needed by many, perhaps most of us humans. It has come to mean that we're seeking relief from an addiction or some behavioral abnormality. We need to get back to who we once were. We need to get healthy, again. We lost our way, blinded by darkness or disbelief or depression or illness. We need to reclaim and reprogram—and we need to change our plastic brains.

I was hit with a surprising question by my brother not too long ago, asking about the time before my fall: Were you depressed? He had come to the hospital to visit me shortly after my fall. I don't remember his visit, only the feeling of a loving presence and I seem to have a memory of the echo of his voice.

In answer to his question, I just said: "Whoa! What?" My wife has asked me that too, in the years after we were married. Me? Mister Happy-go-lucky? Mister eager to shoot the shit or talk it? Mister Life of the Party? Oh, well . . . bingo! Mister life of the party who lived to party and if there was no party, I would make one. Sometimes even alone, just me and a martini. I savored the flavor, of course, but I *loved* the effect. I suppose I was ever seeking relief from—I know this sounds childish—boredom. I just wanted to have fun. On August 14, 2012, I naturally had a cocktail in the afternoon, just an innocent little cocktail (I'm sure more like a couple, and probably strong ones). I did not get behind the steering wheel. I looked out the window and noticed an animal sitting on a tree branch. It was a black animal. It was small enough to be a cat—it was our cat, that damned cat for which my wife had been looking and calling every night for the past couple of nights, now just sitting there, serene. I walked outside and wondered if it could see me coming? (Much later, I learned the cat stayed put. A friend of our family who lives down the road climbed the maple tree the next day or so and simply shooed down the cat. He didn't need a ladder. Ethan has experience as a seasonal logger and carpenter, so kind of knew his way around climbing. Thanks, my friend. And, anyway, I never liked heights.

In my internal intrigue about recovery, note that I don't rush to mention drug therapies, for myself or for recovery in general. I have no experience with recovery drugs such as benzodiazepines. They modulate the brain, of course, and relieve anxiety and are palliatives to addictive behaviors, undoing or preventing the work of glutamates from firing synapses or inhibiting the work of the amygdala (from which fear and anxiety flow), or facilitating or inhibiting serotonin production.

I prefer to think about Earth energy and how we, as electrochemical beings, can channel that or be receptive to it, for our betterment. This involves management of interior space, the function of our brains.

4

THE LOVE OF CAREGIVERS

After my release from the rehab hospital in autumn 2012, an emotional weight was on me. It wasn't caused by my own needed cognitive recovery; no, I was ready to charge into that "training"—my desire to return to my former self was an unbridled motivation. I was troubled by the uneasy memory that my father had Alzheimer's disease. It occurred to me: Would I be facing struggles similar to his? I was in my forties, by profession a communicator, and now my speech and expression were slowed and my thinking and reasoning were cloudy. My processing was much slower, I knew that. Was that how he felt? He was in his early seventies, a retired schoolteacher who moved with my mom (also a retired schoolteacher) to Florida in 2001 so they could begin their retirement in earnest. That never quite took root, as about four years later tests confirmed early onset of Alzheimer's.

I had been with my father a couple weeks before my fall, during my mother's hospitalization for yet another knee surgery. It was her fifth or sixth major knee surgery in three decades, this time for a dislocated artificial knee joint. I was my father's primary caregiver the week I was in South Florida, driving him to the hospital to see my mother, shopping at Publix, doing the laundry, and preparing our meals. I liked being alone with my father and felt I was contributing to his wellness. During the day, he didn't demand much and in the late morning he only needed quiet so he could nap; it allowed me to open my Macbook and keep pace with marketing communication work for the school. But what was he dealing with?

As his son, I was sad watching him sitting inert, placid—or was that vacant? What was going on in his brain? Outwardly, he was the same man I had known my entire life. Now, at times, he just wasn't there. What was going on in his interior space? I was sorrowful and, though I was aware this could be a genetic disease, I didn't stop to think about how my brain might be affected by aging or what might befall me. I was sad for my father, my hero. I wanted him to be happy and comfortable and was relieved that he, at least, wasn't suffering from some debilitating pain, as I knew my mother's knees caused constant pain. I would ask how he was, and he'd simply say, "I'm okay." This was the man who raised me, I loved him, and I wanted to express that love so he would feel it and be reassured and assuaged. I wanted him to at least *feel* that everything was okay, whatever was happening in and to the function of his brain. Of course I wanted him to get better. But also, I wanted him to be at ease. He was through working, after teaching for almost forty years—I wanted him to enjoy retirement in South Florida. We hadn't done enough saltwater fishing on the South Florida flats; we should be holding our fly rods, wading an Atlantic Ocean flat off Key Largo and casting for tailing bonefish! He had no desire to fish, really didn't even think of it. Plus, we were worried about mom; I saw that he was, too.

He was aware of my mother's medical situation and remembered why she was in the hospital but when he wasn't napping he was restless or even impatient or agitated and didn't seem to know what to do with himself when visiting my mother's hospital room. We'd stay for a couple of hours, and then leave my mother to sleep. I stayed in Florida a few extra days to prepare for my mom's discharge, rearranging the house a little to aid her ease of movement, as she was on crutches and would be using a walker.

A couple of months later, I was facing cognitive recovery, just released from the hospital myself.

My wife became my caregiver the moment she found me unconscious on the lawn after my fall. She was incredibly strong throughout my hospitalizations and medical care; because I have no memory from that time, I can only intuit how strong she was. The spouse to whom you've pledged your life, with whom you've had a child, is found on the lawn one summer's afternoon; a 911 call is made, and then the unconscious spouse is packed into an ambulance, rushed to an emergency room, taken by helicopter to a higher-level intensive care unit, and put under observation for a serious brain injury. This in a span of about half a day. Next comes the waiting—for something, anything, to happen. But little does happen. Only sporadic moments of some sign of return to life—a brief focus in the eyes, an uttered word, still unintelligible, maybe a promising smile. Or is that a grimace? When I ask her about it, she says she doesn't want to talk about it. What can you do, she says, other than get on with life? I wasn't aware of the unfolding drama—the trauma occurred and I was aware of nothing. For that reason, I am an unreliable narrator about those weeks of my life. I don't remember, and any flashes of memory might be the work of imagination and the events I'm conjuring never happened at all. I don't know. I'll never know.

Robin told me: "The day it happened, when you got to Dartmouth-Hitchcock, they took an evaluation and decided they didn't need to bore holes in your skull, the pressure wasn't that bad." I fell on Tuesday, and by Thursday my wife wrote in a notebook "no neuro change." She also wrote: "Clinically, no better, no worse." She told me that over the next couple of days she accepted the reality of our family's situation: "You were on disability from work and I recognized we could get by on that for awhile. I decided I wasn't going to dwell on this—you know, I was going to deal with it as the doctors said more." A few days later, when a neuro doctor showed Robin my charts and an MRI of my brain, she wrote "bleeding and damaged throughout, even the untrained eye can see the large spot on the left lobe, controlling speech function, comprehension, and writing."

She later told me: "Basically, on the MRI all I saw was black from the blood and bruising, especially the area of the brain devoted to writing and speech. At that time, you had pneumonia, so that was a concern. You were on anti-seizure medicine. You were in a low-consciousness state—whenever you were conscious they had to tie you up because you would try to get up. They were working with you to see what level they could get out of you. But the doctors wouldn't give you a prognosis; they qualify everything saying, 'Everybody's different.' We talked with social workers who said they would get you into rehab, we had a couple options. First of all, we had to work with the insurance company to see where you could go. But frankly I didn't want to take [our son] Teagan out of preschool," Robin told me.

One of those options was moving me to a rehab hospital near where Robin grew up (and where her parents and sisters and their families lived) in Worcester, Massachusetts; Robin's mother thought that might be a good idea as Robin would benefit from family support. "If you were going to go to Worcester, we would have to go, too. So that's why I say I didn't want to take Teagan out of school," Robin added.

Our son handled the situation with fortitude well beyond his four years, at that time. "Teagan was pretty resilient," Robin said. "He didn't see you early on in the hospital, he wasn't traumatized in any way. I think he handled it well." I learned from my mother-in-law that she made a deal with our son—telling him the family all had jobs to do and his job was to have as much fun as he could staying at my in-laws' house on Cape Cod, with his cousins, so I wouldn't have to worry about him as I was getting better.

I'm not suppressing or repressing recollections—my brain simply was not making or recording memories at this time. I had no consciousness, in the Freudian sense that consciousness is our waking awareness. My eros was active, I was respiring, my heart was beating, and I was eating. Thankfully, I don't remember soiling the sheets or the sputtering and gurgling sounds that were my attempts at speech.

"You were awake then, you were looking around," Robin told me, "but maybe your brain wasn't there. When your brother Tim came to Dartmouth-Hitchcock, we had you outside in a wheelchair and you were speaking to him. You started talking fake German. And you peed in a garbage pail and you said, 'A little maintenance, please.' So you had words. That was funny—you were kind of cocky," Robin said.

I showed signs of recovery, smiling at her and telling her I loved her. Thank God I *did* tell her I loved her, particularly after she was counseled on long-term care options for me. I wouldn't be a danger to her or anyone else, probably, the doctors and social workers said; but I would need full-time care and I wouldn't be the man she married eight years earlier. My mother-in-law Gerry told me I always responded to Robin, or to her voice.

"A doctor told me, 'You should be prepared to care for him 24-7 when you get him home.' I felt like someone punched me in the gut. That was the first time somebody said something like that. I knew insurance wasn't going to pay for 24-7 care—it was going to be me doing it. They were concerned about you walking up and down the stairs—I mean, you were putting toothpaste in your hair at that point," Robin said. This is what my wife had to face—her forty-four-year-old husband, peeing in garbage cans and shitting the bed. Very possibly the man she married would never be seen again.

I was incredibly fortunate—again, blessed!—to have such a loving helpmate, my wife, Robin. I was also fortunate to have married into a medical family, as her mother Gerry and her sister Cindy are both nurses and made sure I was cared for in the weeks after my accident. Gerry said she was there during my early hospitalization to help keep me comfortable and support me in any way possible. She pitched in to help the nurses whenever she could and however she was needed. Gerry and Cindy were advocates for me, as was Robin, who kept notes of all that the doctors told her about my situation. "It was day by day, really," said Gerry. "At that point we didn't know what your recovery would be and we didn't want to think too far ahead, because we didn't know what that might involve." I was restrained for much of that time and Gerry was worried that I might develop bedsores. A pad was placed under me and I didn't. "It's not easy for family. I wanted to look at you and just know that you felt comfortable." At times I was perfectly appropriate, such as when we were watching tennis together on television, but then I would get agitated. Thankfully, I wasn't aggressive or violent. (Still, the compassion came with conflicted emotions because of my reckless and stupid actions on the day I fell.)

In addition to her medical experience, years earlier Gerry had a stroke so she understood brain matters and cognitive challenges such as aphasia, while Robin's father John had had a non-Hodgkin's lymphoma scare a couple of years before. They are wonderful, loving people, truly a second nuclear family. They had to watch their eldest daughter, forty-three years old, be strong in this reality of trauma and shoulder all the responsibilities of our family without knowing if she would have a functional spouse for support in the future. And my mother- and father-in-law helped care for their four-year-old grandson, too, keeping his attention away from my medical condition. My parents and siblings all got regular updates from my incredible wife.

My brother, Tim came to see me as soon as he could at Dartmouth-Hitchcock in August—or so I've been told. I've seen the photo of him pushing my wheelchair and though I'm sitting in the chair, I wasn't there. Except I do have a memory of an echo of his voice, which perhaps was him whispering to me or reading me the newspaper or simply talking to me? I don't know.

I was transferred from the critical-care hospital in New Hampshire to a rehabilitation hospital in Vermont, about one hundred miles away. I had been without consciousness for about three weeks. Several days later . . . I woke up for good—my amnesia lifted, my memory switched on, and my brain resumed function, slowly.

Robin said: "Your acute rehab was three hours a day. Your therapy was speech, physical, and occupational. And then you had to take a nap. I didn't always know what they were doing to try to trigger a response from you, and they didn't always go to the trouble of telling me. You were supposed to come home on September 12, and they delayed you. I was nervous and I remember thinking 'There's no way you're ready to come home.' I guess they had to get permission from the insurance company to keep you." Gerry and her friend Candy visited me and were astounded by how quickly I was coming back and following their conversations and even participating in the back-and-forth. However, nothing was immediate and recovery happened gradually, day by day. Every therapy session, every day, some little part of cognition might pop up—like recognizing the mathematics signs, or remembering some memory from my college years, or being struck by some deadline looming (though already passed) at work. I had the nagging feeling I was forgetting something important, that strange nervous foreboding that I'd previously had in dreams. The feeling of foreboding was a sensation of missed deadlines, as I was attuned to deadlines from my career in publishing.

I had lots of "thinking of you" and get-well-soon cards sent from extended family, friends in the community, and colleagues, and Robin put them in my hospital room; seeing how concentrically love reached me was moving and inspiring, almost dizzying. The heartfelt and sincere messages in the cards, really an outpouring of love, helped trigger memories and warm feelings. Though, at that time, I did not realize the extent of my head injury; I was confused and disoriented. I kept the cards and still look at them and I am so appreciative.

When I was released, I had a solitary focus: to get back to work. "You were gung-ho about going back to work, but I didn't want you to. I think that's what you said about it being like graduation—the first step was getting out of the hospital and then the next step for you was going back to work. You pushed it. I said you didn't need to and I didn't want you to. Your doctor wanted you to take more time, but you wanted to go back," Robin said.

Returning to work became my overriding goal—this, to me, meant returning to normal life. I took a neuropsychological evaluation and I passed. I was in touch with the human-resources director at the school at which I worked and the administration accepted that I was welcome to come back. And so in January, I did.

Robin said she was worried that if I went off disability—she knew I had deficits—what if I lost my job? Then "we'd have nothing," she said.

I ask her now: Did you feel we'd have a hard time as a family? "I wasn't worried about it—until you started pushing to go back to work, and then I didn't know what would happen. I didn't have a lot of time to sit back and think *Oh, my God.* I figured we'd reel in some expenses, and I'd probably sell your car because you wouldn't be driving. I always had support from family and friends," she said.

Soon after my release from the hospital in September, my younger sister Jennifer came from Northern California for a week. (It was the third time since I've lived in Vermont she's visited me. The first was the day after September 11, 2001, when her flight from New York to California was grounded.) Her loving presence rejuvenated my spirit, as we've always had a right-brain, loving-kindness friendship. My memory from that time is still shaky; I know I was slow and unsteady. I remember going for a hike with Jenni on the bike trails up the road from my former house on the side of Burke Mountain. Jennifer and I had lived together in New York City, in a small railroad apartment on 18th Avenue and 8th Street in the Chelsea neighborhood. Spending time with her in fall 2012 brought back jolts of recollections from our New York City days percolating from the hippocampus.

Though I was overjoyed to see her, it was not a joyous occasion for her. She had talked with Robin so knew I was trying to emerge from this cryptic condition none of us understood.

"You were pretty raw. When you see a person you know, completely transformed, it hurts . . . and you were a different person. Maybe it was selfish of me . . . because I went to your house thinking you were going to be okay—and you weren't okay. Your function was much slower, your synapses weren't happening; your whole demeanor was different. Our relationship has always been extremely close, I've felt like in many ways we're an extension of each other, always in step—and it was hard emotionally because you just weren't there. How I could best describe it is I knew you were in there and I just wanted to pull you out, but I couldn't. There were so many instances where I could see you struggle with basic things. And it was such a pleasure for me to be there to help you, because you needed somebody who could comfort you and make you feel comfortable and allow you to make mistakes and not feel like you had to pretend that you were okay."

My sister is right, I was pretending. I wanted to fool everyone into thinking I was okay, I was resilient, I was normal. But at that point, in October 2012, I was not.

My sister is not telling the entire story, either. She was terrified. She expected to see at least some recognizable semblance of her former roommate and older brother. But she did not. She saw a yearning, needing person groping for compassion, time, support, and understanding. At that early stage for the brain-trauma patient, having time to recover is critical.

My sister is successful at a tech company in California; she knows business and how to relate to people. She is compassionate, empathetic, and understanding; she is the best friend you want to have. She wanted to do everything to help me, Robin, and her nephew Teagan. When she was with me—she just watched me, observed, noted what she saw, and did what she felt was right.

"I wanted to have the same person I knew—it's a very hard experience for a loved one because you want to believe that person is going to go back to how we know them but we just don't know if that can happen. It's selfish and selfless, really. We know you're trapped in there and we want to pull you out but there's nothing we can do. I could see you in there, I could see your soul through your eyes and I knew how hard it was. There was nothing that I could do to help you. That's where patience, love, and kindness come into play. There's no doubt that day after day through an experience like this there's going to be some anger and frustration. We're all human and when you can't control a situation like this . . . it's very difficult."

I asked my sister if she had any thoughts about our father's Alzheimer's condition. "With Dad, all I want to do is hold his hand

and spend time with him. I've found in life that the most important thing is spending time with the person. Your experience and his experience have forced me to slow down and have given me guidance and patience and understanding. I look into Dad's eyes, and I see the same person I've always known. There are times I don't even know who he is and it seems absurd; other times, he's the same person. I always try to focus on the positives."

She continues: "With you, I had a finite period of time when I could prepare myself for the week I was there with you. I wanted to help relieve the burden of your wife and spend every minute I could with my nephew." Did she see any hope for me? "The time we picked up Teagan at school and his face just beamed when he saw you and I saw how excited he was, and your face back—it was a moment when I knew you were going to be okay. It was a moment that gave me such hope." Jenni recognized the importance of family support, and she said it's vital to reach out and get as many family members involved as possible. "Just being there and offering any support—just anything— was so, so important."

My parents came to our house from Florida for Thanksgiving, after my wrist surgery. I had messed up the bones in my right wrist and hand—a right perilunate dislocation that required ligament repair and stabilization with K-wires or pins. The right arm bore the most evidence of my fall, as I had no visible injury to my head other than initial bruises. I wore a splint on my arm when they were here. My parents were patient and simply wanted to be with me, Robin, and Teagan. My father played board games with me and Teagan, and we worked together at Word Finder puzzles. I saw some humor in our recovery bubble—the TBI patient, the septuagenarian grandpa with Alzheimer's, and my four-year-old who couldn't yet read or write. We all needed to learn or re-learn, as best we could.

"I didn't know what to expect, I was very apprehensive. I was very scared, I don't think I ever got over being scared," my mother said. "I prepared myself by getting firsthand information from Jennifer and Robin. I think it would have scared me even more if I had read about TBI. Sometimes not knowing is better." I ask her what she noticed when she first saw me: "You didn't have your spark. You took so long in trying to express yourself. You were very hesitant in the words you used and sometimes you struggled to correct yourself."

But she is my mother—she continued: "I was amazed at how well you were doing, I was impressed with the tenacity you had in working on your recovery. I felt guilty that I hadn't been there sooner, to help Robin and to give more support, and to share our love with you and Teagan. I don't think, though, I could have come any sooner. I don't know if I could have."

I asked a tough question: if she saw in my struggles any similarities to what she's seen in Dad? "No, it's different. With him, it's kind of blank. Sometimes his face is just blank and I can't read anything. I never saw that in you. You always worked to express yourself, or tried to anyway. You just wanted to talk and tell us all about what you were going through. You talked a lot and we listened. Sometimes I wanted to ask a question and I would say to myself, *Betty, just shut up and listen.*" She said I wanted to tell them (or try to) how I was feeling and how hard I was going to work to get better. Mom laughed and said, "Sometimes I thought you were a little too optimistic. But you weren't—look what you did! You were back to work a lot sooner than I thought you would be. I have a beautiful memory of you and your dad sharing your birthdays, together." His is November 23 and mine is December 1—fellow Sagittarians.

Now that a couple of years have passed, I asked my wife recently: am I different now?

"Yes," she said without hesitation.

Is it a better different?

"You were kind of day by day for a while. Your brain wasn't working much beyond, 'What's next on the calendar?' You're different, but

I can't pinpoint how. That was always going to be the outcome. They told me to be prepared that you might be incredibly violent and lash out at me, but you never did," she said, and adds with either disappointment or as a playful jab: "But now you don't have a sense of humor."

The anxiety, the doubt, the disappointment, the frustration, the anger—that added up to a different kind of trauma for Robin. Caregivers feel the traumatic circumstance of the patient—and everyone needs time to heal.

Robin concluded about the medical and clinical care I received: "Rehab is amazing. The rehab people were wonderful and I think they did a great job. But we can't dwell on your brain injury for the rest of our lives."

Nope, I don't intend to dwell on my brain injury—only to appreciate for the rest of my days the new consciousness I have, and my ever-increasing knowledge of brain function and awe for the magical, miraculous organ that anchors our nervous systems.

5

NEUROPLASTICITY

Plasticity is the mutability of the brain. Neuroscience is determining that although our genetics contribute much to who we are, our neurological circuitry is not formed completely or definitively at conception and we establish our behavior as we live—we live and we learn, quite literally. Learning, it can be said, is the accumulation of applied experience. The concept of neuroplasticity is that the brain is not hardwired and changes its pathways—its manner and order of functioning and causing function—to reveal changeable behavioral outcomes (hearing, speaking, laughing, moving) that make us each unique individuals, dictated to a great degree by our personal experiences, which change over time and so the applied performance of the brain changes throughout our lives—we react based on past actions. The brain's immediate intent is carried through—synapses fire and we act—so long as we're physically able to do so. In this way, mind coordinates body. The brain moves us to action.

One way to look at neuroplasticity is that you change your mind about something and want to reorient your behavior, so your thoughts reorganize the way the brain achieves functions and you change behaviors that have become habituated or almost seem innate or inborn. The brain is not fixed, scientists now know. So by *wanting* to change, you *can* change. The brain will open up pathways, and help you to think, reason, and act in new ways.

A twelve-step recovery program is an example of this. By talking about experiences, sharing them openly and honestly with others who have likely lived through similar experiences—and doing this anonymously, so you won't feel judged—you can forge new ways of living because your brain is forming pathways leading to new behaviors. You can see and smell the addictive substance (alcohol or drugs), but you no longer crave the sight and odor of it. You are no longer dependent on having to consume it to achieve a specific craved effect (again, in your brain). You can come to think instead, *I don't need that* which may lead to *why would I want that, that's wrong, that's shameful*. I'm not recommending finding and embracing shame or guilt, but those emotions can be strong catalysts in wanting to change.

In the book *The Brain That Changes Itself* by Norman Doidge, neuroscientist Paul Bach-y-Rita is quoted as saying, "We see with our brains, not our eyes," which seems a simple statement but sets up the understanding that the brain processes or channels sensory information to the best benefit of the brain's owner—the heavy bearer who goes with it. This is the basis of plasticity. The example given in the book is about how a blind person "sees" with a cane because the brain decodes sensory information gathered by the hands to make directional decisions.

There are dozens of anecdotal examples of similar altered brain functions in Doidge's book, including an example of a woman born only with a right hemisphere of the brain, yet she has functions thought only possible by the brain's left hemisphere, like speech and language, which are being produced in her right hemisphere. Doidge says in a "normal brain each hemisphere helps refine the development of the other by sending electrical signals informing its partner of the activities, so the two will function in a coordinated way."

Brain cells that "fire together, wire together" is the phrase used by neurological experts, courtesy of the work of Donald Hebb and what is called Hebb's Rule and leads to an exploration of Hebbian plasticity. The basic premise is that individual synapses activate associated neurons and together the chain-reaction synapses combine to cause an impulse or effect. This is a type of synaptic domino theory, in other words.

The book *Synaptic Self* by Joseph LeDoux delivers an easy-to-understand accounting of these Hebbian findings and corollaries. The book helps explain who we are and who we become over time and how that happens. "The existence of a self is a fundamental concomitant of being an animal," LeDoux writes. Not all animals are self-aware, he further points out. Humans are, and perhaps that's what it means to be human—to be aware of the self and our relation to others and to objects. The brain retains our experiences and calculates a reaction to stimulus—desire, fear, apprehension, love—and we embrace, cower, withdraw, swoon. Similarly, the brain changes all the time. If the connectivity—nerve cells, dendrites, synapses, chemical exchanges, axons—that results in speech is interrupted, that interruption is often temporary until the brain detours some of these processes into a new pathway. Speech still results, it just happens through changed circuitry in the brain (or changed neurocircuitry).

The school of synaptic theory began with Santiago Ramón y Cajal, according to LeDoux. Synapses are the living currents of neurological activity, forming our personalities, which come from the reactions instantaneously calculated in the brain. Even to *not* react is a reaction, isn't it? To decide to climb a ladder on a summer's afternoon is incontrovertibly an idea leading to action. Our decisions surely prompt dissenting opinions or counter-decisions. That's what "thinking it over" means. Many people make decisions, commit, and don't look back. Others, like me before I climbed that ladder, turn over the thought, letting it ping through the neurocircuitry like a rock in a tumbler. Well, that's how sharp edges are smoothed, I used to think in a positive way about my internal monologue or inner voice that was constantly speaking to me. I made better decisions because I was always looking at all the angles, so to speak, and weighing all the options and outcomes. But then my internal monologue became relentless and nattering, and my goal-oriented effort in life turned toward finding internal quietude and relief.

There is some debate about the duration of plasticity and how long it is actively possible in the brain. The book *Changing Brains: Applying Brain Plasticity to Advance and Recover Human Ability (Progress in Human Brain Research)* does discuss "critical periods" for plasticity. The book mentions that molecular "breaks" can limit plasticity in adults. Some schools of thought say that so-called cellular plasticity only happens for the first couple of years of life and then we may be less able to create, activate, and assimilate new behaviors. Scientists continue to study this.

Further, neurologists are examining if molecules in neurons change after traumatic brain injury, inhibiting memory and learning as synapses are weakened. An article in the Summer 2014 issue of *The Challenge*, the magazine of the Brain Injury Association of America, written by Coleen M. Atkins, PhD, of the University of Miami Miller School of Medicine, says, "The strength of synapses that connect between neurons is regulated by molecules within the neurons. These molecules are important for the growth of new synapses during learning." The author writes that a molecule known as CREB is crucial for facilitating the process of synapses in the brain. After TBI, CREB can't be activated by neurons, limiting synapses in learning conditions. The article says drugs that target CREB could improve learning and memory after TBI. But perhaps so could neuroplasticity, through deliberate cognitive therapies targeting learning, similar to learning a new language. The brain can change, if we work at changing.

After my head injury and the ensuing cognitive therapy and life introspection, I understand better why I was so completely drawn to a career editing other peoples' words. I have a facility for sharpening thoughts, not necessarily hatching them. I'm a people pleaser, when it comes down to it; I want writers to feel their best about what they are expressing so I help to sharpen and hone the language of their expression. I share in their delight and feeling of success in achievement when the story is finally in print. I am not imperious about the editing. I've learned and retain English grammar and style rules and I abide by them. My neurons brought that stuff to the limbic system and synapses sealed it there. Not all of it—I still write with a dictionary resting on my lap and with resource volumes such as *Chicago Manual of Style* and *The Elements of Style* surrounding my desk—but I remember more about the rules of writing than most people do. I don't retain any amount of trigonometry and very little calculus. I know enough French to stumble through a comprehendible exchange with someone born in the province of Quebec (fifty miles north of where I live). These are some of the elements that make me who I am. My brother (more than a year older than me) and my sister (three years my junior) are different people, though parts of us are the same, the overlaps coming from our experiences growing up in the same house in a small span of time, and our shared DNA. I was three when my sister was born but I do remember a baby coming home. That remains in my cortex, almost fifty years later. LeDoux writes, "To be self-aware is to retrieve from long-term memory our understanding of who we are and place it in the forefront of thought." The conscious and unconscious, in other words, are fundamental pieces of who we are. The two parts of the whole, the Yin and the Yang of Traditional Chinese Medicine, "opposites on a continuum of energy and matter" as the website www.sacredlotus.com tells us.

"The self is not static. It is added to and subtracted from by genetic maturation, learning, forgetting, stress, aging, and disease. This is true of both implicit and explicit aspects of the self, which may be influenced similarly or differently at any one point," LeDoux writes.

Plasticity is science's name for this process. (We have to apply names so we can form understanding, and plasticity is a cool name.) It is a miracle quality—particularly in the sense that we call the unexplainable miraculous. Years or decades or centuries from now, as a species we'll undoubtedly know better how it all works, what chemicals combine

or energy comes into contact to form the thoughts that lead to physical actions. This is the basis of human beauty, to me. It is certainly in the
eye—or within the optic nerve, traveling along retinal ganglion cells—of
the beholder. We don't have to dwell on knowing or not knowing how
it all works. We can delight in the miracles within us and discover more
and apply names to the newly discovered processes. The beauty too is
that the learning linkage is much like "fire together/wire together." As
we learn more about the brain we build on the acquired knowledge and
continue to improve our understanding of who we are as *homo sapiens*
and how and why we operate in the ways in which we do.

To be writing this book and to be able to still think in such a
way that can encourage humanistic discovery is exciting. The Kena
Upanishad, the sacred Vedic text, begins "Who sends the mind to
wander afar? Who first drives life to start on its journey? Who impels
us to utter these words? Who is the Spirit behind the eye and the
ear?" The book *The Mind & The Brain, Neuroplasticity and the Power of
Mental Force* by Jeffrey M. Schwartz, MD, and science writer Sharon
Begley states, "According to Buddha's timeless law of Dependent
Origination, it is because of volition that consciousness keeps arising
throughout endless world cycles." I was excited to read this, and particularly the connection between Buddhism and the word volition,
which means the power to choose or exert one's will—and how this
relates not only to Buddhism and mindfulness, but to quantum phys-
ics, as the authors share in the book.

The word quantum, to me, connotes strange and unexplained phe-
nomena. But perhaps I'm misunderstanding its use. In actuality, the
definition means "a fixed, elemental unit, as of energy." So volition is a
key word in the above, a definitive word really, as it means to employ
will. In this explanation, we chose to exert volition in fixed, measured
(quantum) ways and that is our freedom of choice, gliding through
neuro pathways. No doubt neuroplasticity accounts for this also.

My nephew John is ten years old (as I write this) and was born with a
malformed left cerebellum—hypoplasia of the left lateral cerebellum.

The obstetrician shared this news with my sister and brother-in-law when the baby was in the womb, as scans showed the reduced physiology of "the little brain," as the cerebellum is called.

My nephew Johnny-B is an active boy, curious and, when he sets his mind to something, determined. His eyes tend to orient up in a dreamy way and when he talks to you he looks away, never directly at you. His speech is about as slurred as mine was when I was recovering from my fall, which means he's difficult to understand, sometimes. I'm incredibly touched by his presence in our lives. He goes about his daily boyish business in a happy-go-lucky manner. The cerebellum regulates motion and balance and when he was younger he didn't like jerky, rocking motion; he became physically and audibly agitated by it. Once I saw him become uncomfortable and then terrified on a carnival ride; he seemed to love the straight-ahead-moving log flume, though, and couldn't get enough of the splashing water (it was a hot July day). His mother said when he was an infant he wasn't comforted by stroller walks or rocking, as most babies are. He loves music and can carry a melody that sounds spot on even though he hums or recites nonce words rather than learning and repeating the lyrics, localizing the melody, pitch perfect. He goes to a special services school and is a buddy of my son, who's three years younger; they play together like cousins do, like good friends. I see brotherly love between John and my son, which is uplifting now that I'm more focused on the brain and my own brain function and aware—so much more aware—of how tenuous our states of being truly are.

Let me say I'm sorry for having thoughts in the past (however unexpressed and therefore secret) that people with evident mental deficiencies were somehow regressed or less vital or less valuable than "normal" people were. I remember a friend in college joking about an acquaintance "riding his tricycle into a dumpster when he was a kid" as the reason for the acquaintance's slowness and lack of apparent mental aptitude. In its bony shell, the brain is protected against minor dings and its plasticity allows it to reprogram when necessary, but it's not impervious to assaults or traumatic injuries. The brain is largely fibrous (particularly the core mass), but is still in point of fact soft tissue. Next time you think of undertaking physical risks, think of the brain and what possibly could happen. Thanks to neuroplasticity, you might recover with time and excellent care and loved ones helping you. Or maybe you could avoid all that and rather than undertaking the risky business simply be entertained watching a movie or surfing the Internet—or, experiencing the depth and grandeur and verisimilitude of reading a book. The Kena Upanishad also says: "What cannot be spoken with words, but what whereby words are spoken: Know that alone to be Brahman, the Spirit; and not what people here adore." Another translation from the Sanskrit is "What mind does not comprehend, but what comprehends mind, that is Brahman, not what people worship here."

What this means to me: We can change our outward behavior, our thought processes, and indeed our expressed personalities thanks to neuroplasticity. You are never an old dog; you can always learn new tricks. The French might say *Ce n'est pas à un vieux singe qu'on apprend à faire la grimace*. (You can't teach an old monkey to make a funny face.) But people can learn, *mon ami*.

We can change if we desire to, and we truly put our minds to it. We can learn new ways of behavioral living, just as surely as we can learn new languages and by the same repetitive memorization processes, truly. Your brain will adapt to new knowledge and it will embed that knowledge into your memory bank and it will recall those memories so you react and behave accordingly. Rather than being anxious and harried or aggressive, you can instead face a difficult challenge with equipoise and grace and equanimity. We can learn to do that.

Meditation is called "a practice" for this reason. Like athletics, the more you practice, the more skilled you'll become. Of course, the combined meaning is: to do something frequently; and to observe and adhere to, or habituate. This is the perfect description of what meditation can do for us. We can begin to mold and shape our own cognitive functions and reprogram our brains. The neuroscientist Richard J. Davidson of University of Wisconsin-Madison and the Waisman Laboratory for Brain Imagining and Behavior has studied this phenomenon. In *Mindful* magazine in 2014 he wrote,

> It is now widely accepted that the brain is an organ designed to change in response to experience and…in response to training … Research on neuroplasticity has given us a broad conceptual framework in which to place the research on meditation … and what we see is that even short amounts of practice can induce measurable changes in the brain. Our brains are constantly being shaped, wittingly or unwittingly—mostly unwittingly. We tend to be pawns of the forces around us.
>
> Basic neuroscience evidence suggests that small, short periods of practice done many times in a way that can actually be sprinkled throughout the day is a really powerful way to promote enduring change in the brain.

Additionally, he wrote that this area of study is "inviting us all to actually take more responsibility for our minds and our brains." Scientists have embraced this concept in the last three or four decades, as neuroplasticity emerged from hypothesis and theory to clinical fact. Many therapies center on repetitive practice, meditation, and compassion training. Anthony Burgess wasn't far off into the realm of science fiction when describing the "Ludovico treatment" aversion therapy Alex received in *A Clockwork Orange,* agonizing though it may have seemed. In reality, in neurological and cognitive terms, pathways can be created to elicit certain human behaviors in much the way Burgess's fiction predicted.

Davidson conducted brain research using Matthieu Ricard, a Buddhist monk, as a subject. He monitored brain waves after asking Ricard to meditate on "unconditional loving-kindness and compassion," according to a story in *Wired* magazine called "Buddha on the Brain." Davidson observed powerful gamma activity, which is indicative of intense, focused thought, in the electroencephalography (EEG) output. Other studies on Buddhist monks showed gamma waves thirty times as strong as those from students (used as a lay control group). It would seem the monks were expressing their minds in an intensely focused manner. They'd had a lot of practice in this.

In *The Brain That Changes Itself*, author Norman Doidge describes love as "a period of heightened plasticity, allowing (two brains) to mold to each other and shape each other's intentions and perceptions." Doidge recounts experiences of his therapy patients mapping new pathways toward recovery. We learn in the book that the human cortex alone has thirty billion neurons (and the brain has more than 100 billion, it's estimated) and that accounts for "one million billion synaptic connections." Doidge quotes scientist Gerald Edelman as writing, "If we considered the number of possible neural circuits, we would be dealing with hyper-astronomical numbers: ten followed by at least a million zeros." Doidge continues: "These staggering numbers explain why the human brain can be described as the most complex known object in the universe, and why it is capable of ongoing, massive microstructural change, and capable of performing so many different mental functions and behaviors."

Plasticity, Doidge writes, "introduces new biological brain structures in individuals by non-Darwinian means." When people read, Doidge writes, several parts of the human brain are at work. The joy of reading, indeed!

There are physiological cognitive building blocks, in other words, and as the parts or modules of the brain connect and integrate, new functions or behaviors result. Again, as we live, we learn and we grow. Wire together and fire together, to be sure.

Examples that bear this out are seen time and again in studies of individuals who are blind or deaf and develop stronger abilities in a module of the brain to compensate or overcome the lost sense. "Change in one brain module ... leads to structural and functional change in another brain module," Doidge writes. One sense begins to compensate for a lesser or absent one—the hearing of a blind person can be more acute than in people who see and hear.

This is neuroplasticity, which can help us change our behaviors. The same way this process contributed to my recovery following traumatic brain injury.

6

ATHLETICS AND OTHER RISKS

My home state of Vermont has concussion guidelines for elementary and secondary-school adult personnel—intended primarily for coaches and athletics staff—"to assist schools in taking reasonable steps to prevent, and to minimize the effects of, school athletic team-related concussions," the guidelines read. These were in effect for the autumn 2011 season, the year I coached junior varsity boy's soccer in the Vermont Metro high school league. Soccer was administered, as all high school sports are in Vermont, by the Vermont Principals' Association (VPA), which is responsible for ensuring that coaches receive training in federal guidelines for concussion management from the Center for Disease Control. We coaches were required to watch a video and review an online program called "Heads Up: Concussion in Youth Sports." Every school is required to follow the state law that "requires that schools educate their coaches, their youth athletes, and the youth athletes' parents and guardians regarding the prevention and mitigation of concussion-related injuries."

We coaches had to understand the dangers student athletes faced on the playing fields and how to recognize both a concussion and its effects. Having been a college athlete, I felt I was aware of this, and my co-coach of the JV team and I were tested on our preparedness when a player had a head collision and had to sit out a game and see a doctor for an examination. We followed the guidelines; we put the protections in place; the system worked as intended; the player was okay.

Injuries happen in sports—in high school, I broke my leg playing soccer during my senior year resulting from an opponent's slide tackle. Had the player also followed through into my body and head, I could easily have suffered a broken arm or a concussion. The extrapolation is deliberate: A broken leg is obvious because the leg is swollen and discolored and the recipient complains of pain; a concussion is often invisible and has no evidentiary accompaniment, except maybe a bump or a cut. The tissue effects are inside the skull and nowadays because the result includes the player being restricted from competing, the student won't always share how they're feeling after the impact. They might downplay or underreport it. Lack of awareness of the potential dangers of concussions—the cognitive struggles and even temporary mental impairment, to say nothing of the long-term risks that we aren't completely sure about—means it's likely a teenage player probably won't voluntarily take themselves out of play. We're dealing with kids who feel they're invincible—high school or younger students aren't thinking about their futures.

The Vermont concussion guidelines include these points:

- The Centers for Disease Control and Prevention estimates that as many as 3,900,000 sports-related and recreation-related concussions occur in the United States each year.
- Continuing to participate in athletic and recreational activities with a concussion or symptoms of a head injury causes children and adolescents to be vulnerable to greater injury or even death.
- Despite the existence of recognized return-to-play standards for concussions and other head injuries, some children and adolescents in Vermont with a concussion or symptoms of a head injury are prematurely permitted to participate in athletic and recreational activities, resulting in actual or potential physical injury or death.

The "death" warnings are certainly troubling, but not by any means exaggerated. Coaches are encouraged to remove a player from competition if the player is thought to have a concussion based on an observed or reported head impact or behavior or symptomatology (confusion, imbalance, dizziness, nausea) indicating a concussion. The guidelines point out that the situation is then "a medical decision" not a sportsmanship or a moral one.

The truth is, doctors can't predict the long-term impacts of concussions. Sufferers of concussions seem predisposed to more concussions—some doctors warn that those who suffer a concussion are up to six times more likely to have another—meaning that apparently if you have one and feel the effects, each subsequent head impact can cause a similar or worse effect. Perhaps your understanding of how a concussion will affect you is lost each time you have one. (Here's hoping you'll never have to face or consider this for yourself or your loved one.)

I talked with a friend who had what appeared to be a concussion in high school and then suffered the effects of post-concussion syndrome for years. In the fall of his senior year in high school, in September a couple of weeks into the semester, Parker was president of and first in his class, figuring out where he was headed to college— he had a lot on his plate.

I was at football practice and I was lined up against a teammate in an open-field tackling drill, where we're ten yards apart and he's either going right or left and you have to tackle him. I hit him square, and we both did everything correctly, and his knee came up and hit me under the jaw. It was effectively like getting a huge uppercut. I didn't black out, didn't lose my memory, knew all the answers to the questions—knew who I was, where I was, what day it was, how many fingers they were holding up. But I just didn't feel right. I knew something was wrong.

He began having severe headaches, and found he couldn't read because the words would seem to move across the page. He had his eyes examined and biologically they were fine. But there was no confirmation that the eyes were functioning properly together. He felt, all day, like he was hung over. All he was focused on, at the age of eighteen, was "how can I feel okay, today."

He had an MRI, saw a neurologist, tried alternative therapies such as acupuncture and massage and osteopathy—anything that might help his family arrive at an answer for the condition. The neurologists recommended that it would take time. He worked with a behavioral ophthalmologist to retrain his eyes to work together. He took a gap year in Greece and traveled through Europe, which helped him think *I'm still smart, I can still do this.*

Through an environmental experiential learning program that year back in the United States, he earned the necessary credits to graduate from high school. He tried college, but his headaches came raging back. After a fishing trip on which he met a fly-fishing outfitter, he moved West to guide fly fishers and work in a fly-fishing shop, in Idaho. Next, he started taking college classes in Missoula, Montana. He could read and do the work—"it was a great way to give me the confidence that I could go to school again." He finished college at George Washington University, and didn't have further headache problems. He got an internship at a financial firm, and now works for that firm.

"I find that now, I can function at a very high level. I don't have issues reading, or sitting in front of a computer screen doing spreadsheets all day, but I'm not someone who gets a lot of joy out of reading. Sitting down and reading a book is not enjoyable for me, because my eyes still get tired. I rely a lot on talking and conversation, versus reading." Ever the optimist, he continued: "The injury led me down a very circuitous path, to where I am today. It was a painful and hard thing to go through, but the opportunities it led me to and how it changed my perspective on life, I would never give up. I got so many more positives out of the whole thing, rather than negatives." This was an isolated head injury—post-concussion syndrome—sustained in high school football practice. He recovered, but it took years. He now has a wife, three daughters, and is thriving at his financial-services firm.

At the college level, the NCAA released concussion guidelines in July 2014. They offer the definition of concussion as "a change in brain function following a force to the head, which may be accompanied by temporary loss of consciousness, but is identified in awake individuals, with measures of neurologic and cognitive dysfunction."

College athletes are also less likely to volunteer disclosing their injury, perhaps, as they may be on athletic scholarships or as burgeoning adults will not admit to debilitating injury or perceived disabilities. We also must consider the "indestructible" feeling that comes with youth—in fact, the report cautions that athletes "may underreport symptoms and inflate their level of recovery in hopes of being rapidly cleared for return to competition."

The report concludes that education about concussions is an important element so that athletes understand the risks of competition. Important too is the development of a baseline evaluation that can be used for comparison following a concussion. The NCAA's chief medical officer Brian Hainline stated that about 90 percent of NCAA schools currently record baselines. This might include brain injury/concussive history (if it's happened once, the injury will likely be more serious the next time), symptom evaluation, cognitive assessment, and balance evaluation. Biomarkers, through MRIs or blood tests, might also indicate an athlete's susceptibility to concussions and brain injury.

The NCAA regulations require the at-risk player to rest and seek experienced concussion-management treatment. Returning to academics is addressed also: like return-to-play, the NCAA mandates cognitive rest and gradual return to schoolwork, as tolerated by the player.

I applaud the use of the word "individualization" in the report cited above, acknowledging that each brain injury is personal and that there are no blanket diagnoses or rote treatments. Eventually, this attention could lead to an interschool database in which all 1,100 NCAA member schools can review concussion histories and progressions—if

Health Insurance Portability and Accountability Act (HIPAA) regulations allow. This could involve cooperation with the Department of Defense for a wide-sweeping concussion database possibly showing links between head injuries and long-term brain damage.

"NCAA schools have placed a priority on improved concussion management, but we still have many unanswered questions in this area," said NCAA President Mark Emmert in a published report. "We believe in the incredible potential of this research. Student-athletes will be first to benefit from this effort, but it also will help to more accurately diagnose, treat and prevent concussions among service men and women, youth sports participants and the broader public."

The White House has called this an "Educational Grand Challenge" aimed at creating an overall change to the concussion culture in athletics. Two other initiatives are the National Institute of Health's program to measure the long-term effects of repetitive concussions and the National Institute of Standards and Technology examining protective aids and ways to better protect against concussions.

As I was writing this chapter in the fall of 2014, the University of Michigan's administration and the college's president Dr. Mark S. Schlissel came under pressure and were the targets of protests from students and fans following a hit to the Wolverine's quarterback and his subsequent on-field behavior (tripping, weaving, staggering), which indicated a hard hit likely had concussed him. Boos ensued—not directed at the player, but fans seemed to be reacting because he wasn't taken out of the game. The TV color commentator expressed outrage and incredulity that the head coach allowed the player to stay in the game for another snap.

Already, some colleges are putting player protections in place. Football practices have curtailed contact or moved to half-contact and hitting restrictions. This seems to mirror the NFL curtailing hitting during practices. As at the high school level, once a player is observed to have a possible concussion, return-to-play in college is a medical decision. (It has been the policy in the NFL and other professional leagues for some time—that's called protecting your investment in talent.) "There should be no pressure from a non-medical entity like a coach or administrator to get a player back to the game. The tricky part is moving that to really something that's widely practiced," said the NCAA's Dr. Brian Hainline. You can find more at NCAA.org.

If all of the above sounds like "the sky is falling" guardedness (or "pie in the sky"?), maybe that will change soon. A report in 2014 discussed a blood test researchers are using to diagnose brain injuries and thereby preventing injured players from returning to competition. The study report quotes professor of neurochemistry Henrik Zetterberg of the Sahlgrenska Academy at the University of Gothenburg (Sweden) as saying, "Concussions are a growing international problem."

Indeed, concussions were a much-discussed topic during the 2014 FIFA World Cup soccer tournament in Brazil. An Associated Press report pointed out that, in the World Cup final match, German midfielder Christoph Kramer had to be helped off the playing field and couldn't remember details from his collision with an Argentinian player. "Clearly if there is protocol (to guard against concussion), it isn't being followed," the report quoted Chris Nowinski as saying. He is with the Concussion Legacy Foundation (formerly the Sports Legacy Institute or SLI), based in Massachusetts, an organization with the mission of "solving the concussion crisis by advancing study, treatment, and prevention of the effects of brain trauma in athletes and other at-risk groups." They are affiliated with the Center for the Study of Traumatic Encephalopathy at Boston University, which in turn studies the long-term effects of repetitive brain trauma, with a focus on degenerative brain disease Chronic Traumatic Encephalopathy (CTE), also called punch drunk syndrome or *dementia puglistica*. SLI (now the Concussion Legacy Foundation) began a certification program called Hit Count, which uses a device that measures and counts impacts that occur in sports in which the brain is at risk. Concussion Legacy Foundation continues to promote awareness of counting hits in contact athletics.

"Most hits are unnecessary and occur in practice. By utilizing Hit Count certified products as a teaching tool for coaches and a behavior modification tool for athletes, we can eliminate over 500 million head impacts next season," said Concussion Legacy Foundation Medical

Director Dr. Robert Cantu. I interviewed Dr. Cantu in August 2014, and he adjusted that estimate higher. "You can reduce the number of hits to the head over the course of a season by a billion," he said, recalculating his previous estimate to include a larger population size. "You can reduce the risk of sub-concussive as well as concussive trauma by reducing the number of hits kids are taking. Maybe they're using their head improperly during blocking and tackling, and we can also see that on videotape," leading to correcting those practices, he said. A company called G-Force Tracker makes the first product to be Hit Count certified. "We don't know the number of hits that people should take . . . over time we hope to be able to develop profiles on how many hits people should take over the course of a month, a year, or a season," Dr. Cantu told me.

(A legal judgment in August 2014 in the so-called O'Bannon antitrust case that may entitle athletes to compensation for the use of their likeness and name could also pave the way for other forms of compensation. Dr. Cantu of the Sports Legacy Institute told me that "the NC2A has insurance programs for their players while they're still in school. But kids who had to leave school due to post-concussion syndrome symptoms, those individuals are without insurance. There should be some kind of workman's compensation for athletes," he points out.)

Similarly, the blood test I mentioned earlier is for traumatic encephalopathy, which can lead to loss of cognitive function and dementia. The substance found in brains of deceased CTE sufferers is a protein called tau, which has also been detected in deceased Alzheimer's patients' brains. Researchers say this blood test could also tell medical personnel the severity of the head injury and the likelihood of long-term consequences.

Dr. Robert Glatter, director of sports medicine and traumatic brain injury in the department of emergency medicine at Lenox Hill Hospital in New York City, said the finding is important. "Identifying a reliable marker that correlates with the severity of brain injury, as well as the recovery, can help track progress and improvements after a concussion, and this can provide an objective measure for safe return to play," Glatter said. "This is a very promising study that opens the door to looking at biomarkers that can help us to provide better care to athletes with concussions," he added. Chronic Traumatic Encephalopathy is associated with memory loss, confusion, impaired judgment, paranoia, impulse control problems, aggression, depression, and progressive dementia, Concussion Legacy Foundation operating as SLI reported.

CTE is gaining lots of attention as society (and the media) scrutinizes players in the National Football League and National Hockey League, particularly cases in which a player or former player committed suicide. One such example was Andre Waters, who played in the NFL for the Philadelphia Eagles and Arizona Cardinals in the late 1980s and mid-1990s, and is on record admitting to memory and impulse control problems. His brain was examined after his death by neuropathologist Dr. Bennet Omalu of University of Pittsburg and evidence was revealed of brain damage likely caused by the concussive impacts of playing football. A news story in *The New York Times* by Alan Schwarz on January 18, 2007, reads "the depression that family members recalled Mr. Waters exhibiting in his final years was almost certainly exacerbated, if not caused, by the state of his brain—and that if he had lived, within ten or fifteen years—Andre Waters would have been fully incapacitated."

The New York Times report goes on: "Dr. Omalu's claims of Mr. Waters's brain deterioration . . . add to the mounting scientific debate over whether victims of multiple concussions, and specifically long-time NFL players who may or may not know their full history of brain trauma, are at heightened risk of depression, dementia and suicide as early as midlife." The associated publicity surrounding the story touched off widespread examination of professional athletes, particularly those in the NFL and NHL, to better learn how they may be endangering their health. Head injuries in the NFL have become a contentious societal topic in the recent past, during the same period in which Marines and enlisted soldiers are returning home from the Middle East wars and military actions with TBI and PTSD.

In an interview with former NFL quarterback Boomer Esiason, I introduced a question about concussions at the end of our conversation, telling Esiason about my fall off the ladder and resulting memory loss and cognitive recovery. His response about concussions (not my fall) follows:

> The more discussion, the better. I like the fact that the NFL is so open about it and so understanding that there is a concern about long-term effects of playing football. There's no two ways about it. Do I agree with all their assessments? Most likely not. But I also understand that we as athletes—me as an athlete—got paid a lot of money to play a game I didn't have to play. Never did one doctor, for any of the teams that I played for, ever put me back on the field before I was ready to go back out there. Whether it be concussion related, ankle related, shoulder related, finger related, knee related. I was never asked to take a numbing shot, I was never asked to take anything to go back on the field, and I got paid a lot of money to play. My life afterwards probably is more successful than my life as I was playing and the reason is because of what the NFL gave me. I will never look at the NFL in a negative light. And if I could do it all over again, I'd be the first guy in line to go play football and put that helmet on and play in front of 80,000 people.

Boomer was friendly, approachable, conversational. He said he had at least five concussions while playing.

Our societal fascination with football as a spectacle capturing our attention through intrigue, drama, fear, and violence is matched by our fascination with extreme sports. Everyone loves a good crash, right? ESPN has made millions exploiting that attention through its X Games. We viewers also appreciate the athleticism required to compete, whether jumping objects by launching off a ramp on a dirt bike or doing a cab 180 or air-to-fakie or Rusty Trombone on a snowboard in an icy half-pipe.

The walls of the half-pipe in competitive snowboarding now tower to twenty-two feet, probably around the height from which I fell off the ladder, though I landed on spongy grass and was cushioned somewhat by my extended right arm but still crashing onto my bare head. One of the most horrific crashes documented in an icy twenty-two-foot half-pipe happened to Kevin Pearce, among the world's top snowboarders heading into the Vancouver Winter Olympics, until he crashed in 2009. He had become the rival of Shaun White for men's snowboard supremacy, particularly in the half-pipe. Pearce was attempting a cab double cork (two frontside diagonal flips with inverted twists) when he caught the edge of his snowboard on the icy wall while descending and slammed into the half-pipe, head first. Kevin was in a hospital for three months and trudged through cognitive and physical recovery; and then, realizing the absence of the high of snowboarding from his life, decided he wanted to ride again. He did, but came to understand (with the help of family and doctors) that he just didn't have the same coordination and athleticism as he did before his injury. He was much better as a commentator than a competitor. You can take in all of this by watching *The Crash Reel*, the documentary about Kevin's traumatic brain injury and recovery. Shaun White won the snowboarding gold medal in Vancouver in. The entire snowboarding community rallied to support Kevin Pearce during his recovery by wearing "I Ride for Kevin" stickers. In some ways, the "I Ride for Kevin" movement at that time helped launch increased awareness of traumatic brain injury.

I find that I'm not as coordinated now, either, after my fall. As a former college athlete, I always considered my coordination one of my strong qualities, perhaps even a quality that separated or differentiated me from others. Not any more. I'm simply clumsy now. I fumble stuff all the time. (I reached for a coffee travel mug this morning and spilled coffee all over the table; not for lack of depth perception, it was simply doddering clumsiness.) I'm constantly on guard about falling again.

I also wanted to snowboard after my injury, I wanted to get back to so-called normal stuff. I'm a recreational snowboarder and have ridden since the late 1990s, giving up skiing to snowboard exclusively and working hard to master the sport, stoked to be surfing the earth and feeling the same physical rush and natural sensation that I did growing up water-skiing. In 2002 alone, I figure I snowboarded more than seventy days at six or more resorts in Vermont, including hanging out at the US Open Championships at Stratton Mountain and watching from the media area on top of the half-pipe, getting pictures of Ross Powers and Kelly Clark at the apex of their amplitude above the pipe. I also watched one of Kevin Pearce's homeboys in the "Frends crew" of snowboarders Luke Mitrani of Vermont competing in the Open half-pipe when he was truly a grommet. I've also been on the steeps of Jackson Hole, Wyoming. I've tried a few tricks in the half-pipe (a much smaller version than today's twenty-two-footer, maybe fifteen feet) and remember once falling hard enough in the half-pipe to have my bell rung. Was that a concussion? Maybe. From the success of *The Crash Reel*, Kevin Pearce and his brother, Adam, founded the LoveYourBrain foudation, whose mission statement is as follows: *LoveYourBrain Foundation is a non-profit organization that aims to improve the quality of life for people affected by traumatic brain injury. We develop programs and experiences that integrate mindfulness and movement to help people protect and nourish the brain. We believe our efforts will lead to a healthy, happier world.*

I have my LoveYourBrain T-shirt (which benefits the LYB foundation) and bought one for my son and my wife. Together, we will love our brains. Kevin was named 2014 National Geographic Adventurer of the Year for his work educating people about protecting, respecting, and loving their brains.

The Crash Reel is a powerful dose of "should I?" and "what if?" as, during its filming, the freestyle skier Sarah Burke died in the half-pipe in Park City (the same pipe in which Kevin fell, spookily enough). Sadly, this type of tragedy is no longer surprising and certainly not shocking. To paraphrase Boomer Esiason, the risks are plain but the money is good and the adulation is voluminous. Olympian Bode Miller's brother, a professional snowboarder, died from apparent seizures likely resulting from brain injury suffered in a motorcycle crash. Chelone "Chilly" Miller was found dead in 2013 in the back of his van, his mobile home, at Mammoth Lakes Ski Area in California. My heart goes out to the Miller family.

Kevin Pearce was wearing a helmet at the time of his crash. He has said that it saved his life. Helmets are rated to protect from impacts the wearer travelling about 14 to 17 miles an hour; after that, the impact of the crash will likely be injurious throughout the body and other vital organs besides the brain may be impacted, resulting in serious injury or death. In a crash, kinetic energy becomes deformation energy and the brain is compressed by the deceleration or sudden stop. The brain slams the skull and trauma results, as brain tissue shears or compresses. The outer shell of a helmet is important, but so is the padding inside the helmet, which cushions the head and brain by absorbing the force, lessening the direct force of the impact (acceleration and deceleration). Helmet styles run the gamut, and most helmets are intended to prevent injuries caused by falls or collisions (with tree limbs or people), similar to bike helmets; however, they won't save you in extreme falls or at high-speed collisions with immovable objects. Most recommendations call for helmets to be discarded after a crash. Football helmets are designed to withstand impacts repeatedly, and at the school level can stay in the equipment inventory for years. Depending on the information source, the recommended safe period or "shelf life" of a football helmet is five to ten years. That's a considerable variance. In 2014, helmet manufacturer Riddell introduced the SpeedFlex helmet, which has an articulated "shell panel" covering the frontal lobe and forehead to absorb or cushion the impact of collisions.

The National Operating Committee on Standards for Athletic Equipment (NOCSAE) board of directors has approved the development of a revised football helmet standard that will require helmets to limit certain concussion-causing forces. Now that we acknowledge that we can mitigate head injuries in sports, and we know how the brain is impacted by collisions (that is, how brain tissue responds), NOCSAE is moving forward with the development of a more comprehensive helmet standard than previously existed. Rotational forces involved in concussions are another factor taken into consideration by NOCSAE. This kind of examination has thankfully just about eliminated skull fractures from football, for example, so new helmet standards may similarly reduce concussion risk.

"While it is unlikely the concussion risk can ever be eliminated from sports, this revised football helmet standard should bring us closer to effectively addressing some of the forces associated with concussions," said NOCSAE Executive Director Mike Oliver, in a press release. NOCSAE Vice-President Dr. Robert Cantu, also of the Concussion Legacy Foundation in Boston, has been driving NOCSAE's focus on concussion research since 1996. "NOCSAE has been focused on sports-related concussions for more than fifteen years, and has funded more than eight million dollars in concussion-specific research since 1996," said Dr. Cantu. "I believe NOCSAE is finally at a point where we can revise our standard to incorporate the science and provide improved protection against concussions."

The revised standard could be implemented soon. "Concussive and traumatic brain injuries can change or end an athlete's life. This horrible reality in sports has driven us for almost two decades to push science for an answer to sports concussion risk," said Dr. Thomas Gennarelli, Emeritus Professor of Neurosurgery, Medical College of Wisconsin in a report. "That work has reached the point where we now have a scientific basis to address this risk through performance standards specific to concussion risk."

Dr. Margot Putukian, Director of Athletic Medicine at Princeton University, has earned a NOCSAE grant to study the effects of head impact biomechanics on short- and long-term neurological status in collegiate men's and women's lacrosse and soccer players. This study will use a new head motion sensor patch from X2 Biosystems to better understand the forces and frequency of head impacts in lacrosse and soccer and to determine the necessity of additional protective equipment. Assistant Professor Dr. Kristen Kucera, University of North Carolina Chapel Hill and the National Center for Catastrophic Sports Injury Research, recently earned a NOCSAE grant to expand research aimed at the epidemiology of catastrophic sport injuries. NOCSAE is an independent and nonprofit standard-setting body that aims to enhance athletic safety through scientific research and the creation of performance standards for protective equipment. It is the leading nongovernmental source for concussion-specific research funding in sports medicine and science.

"NOCSAE funded and supported research has brought us to a greater understanding of the science behind sport-related concussions, but more work is necessary to make sports safer for athletes. NOCSAE has been committed to concussion research for more than fifteen years and will continue making further investments into concussion related research, with the belief we can continue to improve athlete safety," said Oliver.

For more information on helmets and to gain an understanding of which models are recommended for specific risky sports, parents and athletes can look to the American Society for Testing and Materials, the Snell Memorial Foundation, American Academy of Orthopaedic Surgeons, Concussion Legacy Foundation, the U.S. Safety Product Commission (CPSC), Common European Norm, and the aforementioned National Operating Committee on Standards for Athletic Equipment. These are information sources for civilians; the military has its own testing standards for combat helmets and personal armor.

Of course, those engaged in the risky activities give their own opinions, from time to time. Brandi Chastain, who won two World Cups with the US women's soccer national team (you might remember the photo of her on her knees with her arms flexed triumphantly, clad in a sports bra, after the 1999 World Cup), says that kids should refrain from heading a soccer ball.

Young players, those under fourteen, might not have the physical strength to absorb the impact of heading the ball using their necks, the way more mature players have been taught and understand they have to so they can direct and propel the ball as they intend, she told the public-radio show *Only A Game*. "The ratio of the velocity of the ball to the strength in young peoples' necks, it's hard for them to protect themselves. And if we take that variable out and we give it to them when they're ready to be more dynamic and aggressive, the better for everybody," she told the radio interviewer. "I've come to realize that heading the ball as a youngster is not really something that we should encourage." She also talked about her former national-team teammate Cindy Parlow Cone retiring from playing soccer because of post-concussion syndrome. These world-class soccer players are now promoting a program with Concussion Legacy Foundation called Safer Soccer that aims to prevent concussions to youth under age fourteen playing soccer.

Skilled players are taught to head a soccer ball with the forehead or side of the forehead (forward of and above the temple), driving the ball at a glancing angle when directing it with power toward the goal, or pushing it straight out when trying to clear it, on defense. Unquestionably, you feel a header, though not as a head-jarring impact when you snap your neck to drive the ball with the forehead. This seems to go against Newton's third law of motion—for every action, there is an equal and opposite reaction—as the head (or skull) is driving the leather or synthetic ball, not really absorbing the impact. Conversely, I've had many dizzy spells after heading the ball with the top of my head (the crown), and I consider myself lucky in my playing days that I never had a head-to-head collision with another player, or with the goal post.

The air temperature seems to make a real difference with header impacts, too. In cold weather, the ball seems harder, as the leather or synthetic cover is less flexible and air inside the bladder is compressed, I suppose. (I once contested the goalie in a college game on a cold autumn day, and as the goalie drop kicked the ball it struck me in the face; the ball felt like cement, I became disoriented; I had my bell rung, which was probably a mild concussion.) I'm almost six foot, two inches and was good in the air, in soccer parlance. I headed the ball often, when I played. It wasn't my signature strength (like timing volleys was, an act of pure coordination), but I was good at it. But is this a risk that we deem acceptable for our children playing soccer? Alas—it is only a game, as the name of the radio show reminds us.

Since September 11, 2001, and the ensuing War on Terror, the US military has become more vigilant about brain injuries than in previous wars, both suffered from concussive blasts or external forcible impacts such as shrapnel or gunshots—but also from combat trauma.

"They called it Agent Orange sickness, they didn't know how to diagnose it. They're not one hundred percent sure how to treat it," Marine Corps Sergeant Andy said about Post Traumatic Stress Disorder (PTSD), an invisible malady much like Traumatic Brain Injury. Both are suffered by military veterans and are now being fully recognized as menacing and life-changing afflictions.

"I had two tours in Iraq. I was in charge of the Fallujah Development Center," Andy said. He served as a Sergeant in Iraq from 2002 to 2003 and 2006 to 2008, when he was Camp Commandant of Fallujah Development Center. He met the woman who became his wife at a concert in Myrtle Beach in 2004, as she visited her Marine Corps brother. After getting out of the Marines in 2008, he took a job in security and worked that for nine months until "all the people felt like pressure." He became reclusive and "started noticing other things going on in my life." When prisoners clean up the roadsides, they leave behind full garbage bags for later pick up. Seeing a garbage bag at the shoulder of the road caused him to stop on I-94 in Minnesota. "Countless times we saw people get blown up by those bags at the side of the road."

"I didn't think anyone understood what I was going through or what I was thinking. I alienated myself away from everybody, which in turn caused me to lose my job. I swore I didn't need help, I'd get through it on my own. I was having nightmares; the only way I could sleep was to physically exhaust myself. I drove my wife nuts, I would stay up for four or five days at a time, just so when I slept, it was sleep—no nightmares, no nothing. There'd be times when I would wake up my wife, and she said my eyes were open and I'd appear fully awake, but I wasn't. I would be giving her orders, that she needed to get out on post, and about incoming fire, shouting orders to her. Which she didn't understand. That started to put a wedge between me and her, it came to a point where we went through an eight-month separation and I moved out to downtown Minneapolis and stayed in my little one-bedroom apartment and never left."

Throughout the day, in every situation, Andy said he has to process thoughts as a Marine first and then rethink them as a member of everyday society. This "double-processing" is exhausting. Marine training was all about muscle memory taking over, and Andy knows now that he needs to process thoughts another way. "My initial reaction was to process everything as I would in combat, and that was causing a lot of turmoil in my life," he said. Now he has to stop and think: *This isn't a normal reaction.*

If somebody screams in a crowded movie theater, Andy explained, he has to stop and rethink that he doesn't need to tackle them because they might be trying to blow up everyone with a bomb. His wife calls it being Doctor Jekyll and Mister Hyde. He said he has trouble differentiating what happened then in combat from what's happening now. He talks about the man within him. "There's the little man that hides down inside me, and then there's the normal me. And every once in a while, the normal me likes to go down there and poke the little man with a stick; but as long as he's chained up, it's okay," Andy said.

"In January two years ago, I had a failed suicide attempt. I got to a point where my body and my mind and my heart were so exhausted from being in two places at once—with PTSD from a combat situation, you have to process everything twice. Once as a normal, functional, everyday member of society; and whatever caused the PTSD, you have to process it that way, too."

It wasn't a conscious decision to end his life, but was caused by having curiosity about what would happen if he died. He attempted to hang himself in the woods, and "fortunately the branch broke." His daughter was three at the time. He had just moved home a couple of days before, following the trial marriage separation, and afterward he looked at his daughter and his wife sitting on the couch in their home. He realized he needed to go talk to somebody to find out what was causing these feelings. He went to the Veteran's Administration Hospital in Minnesota. "It was a huge wake-up call for me."

He's now 80 percent disabled and is not supposed to be around large crowds of people. He works part-time at a camp in northern Minnesota, doing whatever is needed—the laundry, cleaning the dog kennels, dressing harvested game birds, or straightening up the main lodge. He's supposed to keep stress to a minimum, he's not supposed to do anything that reminds him of combat. He bow hunts, but doesn't carry a gun, and he feels his hunting and sitting in a deer stand is a form of meditation.

"You're alone with your thoughts, there's nothing else in the woods, then you see a squirrel, and you go back to thinking. It might not be the official definition of meditation, but it's the closest I can get. I can process the thought fast or slow, or let it go."

At the VA, he was assigned a counselor and realized that you can't stop the triggers resulting from combat. He began a twelve-week coping program, picking the worst experience from war and going into it deeper every week. He wrote out the experience in week one, week six, and week twelve. It became more accurate and vivid each time. The more that memory came back, the more Andy could deal with it. He was suppressing the memories: "You can't fight an enemy you can't see." But they were unlocked and released while he slept. "You can't make yourself busy when you're sleeping so you can forget about it, you can't drink or self-medicate when you're sleeping, so that's when it would creep back in." In the twelve-week program, he realized with the help of his counselor how dangerous it is to suppress the thoughts and try to hide the traumatic memories from yourself. He said that so many vets, generations apart having fought in different wars with different technologies, have the same exact feelings—PTSD is always there. "The images are different, but it's the exact same scenario."

He also gets support from the Marines with whom he served. His wife Lindsay listens to the stories of what they're going through because it's the same as what Andy went through. "We can talk each other out of our bad spots," Andy said.

The VA has been great, too; he goes once a week and it's a coming-home feeling being with other veterans even though it's a hospital. He takes antidepressants and sleeping pills so he can "function every day like a normal human being. The medication helps, but having someone to talk to who has had similar experiences is so important."

He's not critical of the military, but feels more can be done to prepare military personnel (and their families) for the possibility of facing PTSD. There was a warning discussion on their way back from Iraq, on the transport ship. "As a Marine, you get a weeklong class on driving a car, even though we've been doing that for years before we became Marines. And we spend countless hours on weapons maintenance. Well, our minds are technically weapons too when we're in the Marines, so why don't we spend time on the maintenance of that? They don't teach you how to stop being the war machine that they've created . . . our minds are so complex."

Andy doesn't expect a cure for PTSD, but a brain-function toolbox—techniques for managing and maintaining our minds—can help people cope with traumatic events, he suggests, whether encountered in combat or as first responders, violent-crime victims, or fire and emergency personnel, he continues.

"Once you can function, you can learn to live again; once you learn to live again, you can start enjoying life again. But if you're barely functioning, you're not living." Though not a "counselor-type person," once he started listening to the help and advice of his VA counselor, and how it applied to his life, the more he realized he could overcome PTSD. Once again, because PTSD occurs in the brain—and happens in our thoughts—the affliction is individualized. Talking with Andy makes it clear that individualized treatment is the best course of action, rather than the expectation of a miracle brain-function drug, which at any rate does not exist.

"I want to live my life—not just function, but to live, enjoy what I'm doing, and have a sense of purpose."

7

BRAIN INJURY SURVIVOR STORIES

Sue Shirland, 68 (as of August 2015)
Hometown: Colchester, Vermont
Accident: Trauma in 1990, following a fall off a horse

Sue Shirland is a longtime equestrian (with honors ranging from Horse of the Year at first or second level to National Ranking at the top level, Grand Prix). She owns Down East Farms in Colchester, Vermont. She rides horses and instructs riders.

"In 1990, I went to Florida to compete in dressage to try to make the world-championship team. I really didn't expect to make the team, it was my first time giving it a go. I was long-listed for the Olympic team, in 1989, so it was reasonable for me to compete. I wasn't Tiger Woods, but I could play the game. In Florida, I went to one competition and I won the Grand Prix. We were staying in our motor home on a private farm with the horses," Sue said. She and her husband, Larry, on sabbatical leave from the Business School at the University of Vermont in Burlington, had made the trip to Florida so Sue could compete at the top level of dressage. Dressage is an Olympic sport, and at that time the next Summer Olympiad was 1992 in Barcelona,

Spain. A spot on the World Championship team at that time meant the possibility of Olympic competition.

She doesn't remember the accident, a condition that's not uncommon when brain injury is the outcome. "I was not there when it happened. What I'm told is that I was riding my horse in an outdoor arena. One of the things my horse did best was rein back; he did that beautifully. Apparently, I was doing that and he got his feet tangled up in the sugar sand and he fell, and I guess he fell on me. I don't remember any of this. I don't remember riding that day, or anything," Sue tells me. Sugar sand is the ultra fine-grained sand found primarily on beaches in Florida and parts of the Atlantic Coast and is difficult for people to walk in, much less a hooved and horseshoe-shod, thousand-pound or more horse to trod in. The fact that sugar sand was on the ground of the outdoor arena in Florida was simply bad luck.

"Ande, my groom, was talking to me and something happened and I went quiet and the horse got up and ran away. After that, I'm told she said something to me and there was no response, so she shook me. My breathing pattern changed and became very stressed. Then she remembered you weren't supposed to move someone with an injury; she thought she killed me."

People in attendance called 911 and a helicopter landed across the street. Sue said she was wearing her competition clothes, including a new pair of riding boots that the EMTs cut off her feet—"which I think was a way to find out if I was really unconscious," she said with a laugh. "Although there wasn't any physical sign of injury, I remained unconscious." She went to the hospital in the helicopter.

"I think I was in a coma for about ten days. Coming out of it was gradual, I'd open my eyes a little bit or I'd respond a little bit. I don't remember any of that. They had me restrained and I'm claustrophobic, and I know I didn't like it. My first memory is a vague memory of being on the floor in the bathroom unable to get up and thinking, *Oh shit, I've really blown it now.* I had managed to get up and get out of the restraints in my bed. When Larry came in, in the morning, I had stitches in my forehead."

Larry, upon seeing her fresh wound and stitches, asked the doctors exactly what kind of care they were providing? They told Larry they were monitoring her. Larry said, "Yeah, you're doing that so well she gets loose and falls on the bathroom floor and has stitches in her head."

Larry took Sue home to their motor home. "At that point, I really didn't understand what had happened to me. I remember sitting in lawn chairs and falling over."

Because she didn't remember her fall off the horse, she didn't understand why she was under medical care. She had language problems and that became obvious to her when she was trying to talk with a saleswoman at Sears and the woman couldn't understanding what Sue was saying.

"I could hear myself, it was my first realization that I couldn't talk. It was very upsetting." She didn't begin to understand the breadth of her injuries till about two months later.

The doctors knew she had a brain injury but, in 1990, it was not called a TBI. She doesn't remember having an MRI or CT scan and she can't recall seeing the results of any diagnostic imaging, other than X-rays. "There was no TBI diagnosis. They must have determined somehow that I didn't have a bleed in my head, because they didn't open me up. There was not a mark on me.

"My sense of self was very diminished, though. Another thing I remember about being in Florida: In dressage, there is passage, a slow-motion, elevated trot—it's a lot of energy going up and down—and in my outpatient rehab, I remember looking down at myself doing this weird thing when they asked me to try to run down the hall. It was not running at all. I thought about it a lot. What I was doing was more like passage. *That's just not right*, I said to myself."

Sue told the doctors about this discovery that she was going up and down like passage and that to run she had to change the energy to forward and that she practiced that. "The doctor said, 'You must not make decisions like that for yourself. The old you could do that. The new you must not do that.' For months after that, I couldn't do anything without checking with someone. I was so susceptible. I found a typewritten paper in a coat almost a year later, a folded up piece of paper that read 'Get to know the new you.' It went on at some length about, 'There was a person you used to be, and that person had certain talents and certain skills and abilities and strengths and weaknesses. But that person is gone and you must not try to be that person anymore. Get to know the new you. Discover your new strengths and weaknesses and your new likes and dislikes.'"

She was enraged when she read that and immediately adopted an "Oh, yeah? Watch this!" attitude.

"My muscle memory in general was gone after the injury. I couldn't wash my hair, my arms wouldn't work right. I had to relearn everything. Before I went to Florida, I had been teaching riding to a woman named Nancy Binter in Burlington, Vermont, who is a neurosurgeon. I talked with Nancy on the phone just before we left Florida to come home. She asked me, 'You told me everything, right?' So I told her about the tingling. I tingled everywhere, I told people that all the time but they didn't want to hear it. Nancy said, 'Don't do anything, when you come home (to Vermont) call my office immediately, I want to see you.' I just said 'okay.'"

Sue went to Nancy's office, and she had an MRI. Later, Nancy called and told Sue to come back right away. She had two discs ruptured—"blown badly" is how Sue describes it—in her spinal cord. "You are a whisper away from being a quadriplegic due to severe compression of the cervical spinal cord," Nancy told her.

She had surgery three days later; her neck was fused in two places in the spine.

She tells me this was an injury similar to the one suffered by the actor Christopher Reeves; only his spinal cord was compressed to eight mm, leaving him a quadriplegic. "With the spinal cord, eleven mm is the normal diameter, mine was compressed down to nine," Sue said. "I don't know how much (impairment) was from the head injury and how much was from the spine injury. After the surgery, there was a definite immediate improvement. It was a good two years before I could speak very well. I had to think about what I was going to say.

It was because the muscles wouldn't form those sounds. I could find the words, but my mouth wouldn't say the words," she explained. "I knew the words. I couldn't say them. I tried for months, and I would practice. I tried so hard so say 'baby buggy.' I just couldn't. And one day I was practicing in my car, and I did it! I don't know if that's aphasia or not," she replied to my suggestion that she may have been suffering a speech problem like Broca's aphasia; more likely, it could have been apraxia.

"I did my own therapy," she said, by way of pointing out that medical protocol in the 1990s was not as advanced as it is today. "Therapy never worked me nearly as hard as I wanted to work myself. A lot of my recovery was due to the same things in me that made me a successful dressage rider. You have to have a thick skin, you have to be determined, you have to be willing to deal with setbacks, you have to be able to have priorities, and you have to prioritize and figure out all the little pieces. When somebody said, 'You probably can't do this,' I said, 'Oh yeah? You don't think so, huh? Watch this!' I did ninety-eight percent of my own therapy. I would break things down and work on the pieces, because I couldn't do the big stuff. I would decide I wanted to keep my left foot in the stirrup, for example, and I would work until I could do that. I would find ways around to accommodate what I couldn't do yet, but I began to get confidence that I could."

Her reasoning wasn't affected, but her emotions were. "We all have egos, you might not be a jerk about it, but somewhere inside you, that's your self-worth. I couldn't talk right; I couldn't ride right. Before I was injured, I could ride at the top level. And then I got injured, and I still had all the knowledge, but my body wouldn't do what my brain told it to do. And you don't know if it's ever going to come back. It was totally not fair (to Larry) to be stuck with this inadequate person and he shouldn't have his life ruined by being stuck with me, I thought at the time, because he is an honorable man he would never consider doing something dishonorable. I thought he shouldn't be punished for being a good guy."

"You thought you were worse than you were," Larry interjected into the conversation. "I'm not sure I really thought too much about the consequences. I just watched what happened, day to day. I said, 'This is what it is and if it doesn't get any better, well, I can deal with that.' The one-day-at-a-time kind of thing. After the first couple of weeks, you seemed to constantly improve as time went on. I didn't necessarily see a plateau."

"I was back to riding (in 1990) after the spinal surgery in April, after maybe ten weeks, into June when Dr. Binter said I could begin to ride. I wanted to. It was maybe five years before I would get back to where I'd been. I was so frustrated that my body wouldn't do what it was supposed to do. I could continue to see things changing for at least seven years," she said.

Sue belongs to the New England Dressage Association (NEDA), and about three years after her accident they asked her to be the keynote speaker at the Fall Symposium. "I made quite a production—I had music and slides and a story to tell," she said. Though she wasn't wearing a helmet when she fell, helmets are now required by NEDA.

"I went back to Florida one more time to ride competitively, in 1994. I was fully present. And I decided that I really didn't like it that much. You have to leave everyone at home, and there are politics involved. I think I'm a better rider now than I was then. *Better* meaning—I do a better job. I'm a better teacher. Now, I can tell people when they ask 'How do you do that?' Many top riders can't tell you how they do it—they just do it. Now I can tell people how I do it because I had to reteach myself.

"This is equine therapy, it connects body and brain. I always found joy in the riding and training. But competing was never the most important part; riding was the most important part. As long as I could ride again, I didn't need to compete. Horses are so generous. And you can figure out how to communicate with the horse. I could work on that all day long. It's nice to be able to go to a competition and have that validated. But if I had to choose between riding and competing, I would ride as much as I want and not compete." She still trains, teaches, and competes at the highest level, but has cut back on her schedule. This gives her more time to spend with her dogs—a giant Schnauzer and standard Schnauzers—and Mary the one-eyed cat . . . and, of course, her husband Larry.

Sue identified the three most important factors for those who have suffered head injuries:

1. Don't let the injury define you.
2. Don't let someone else tell you what you can or can't do.
3. Be patient, recovery continues for a long time.

Hannah Deene Wood, 42 (as of August 2015)
Hometown: Jericho, Vermont
Accident: Traumatic Brain Injury, October 2001

Hannah Deene Wood has always labeled herself a humanitarian—caring, loving, reaching out to others is what fills her up the most. Her motto is "As the giver, I am the receiver." After graduating from University of Vermont, she managed a skateboard shop in Burlington, working every day and becoming a second "mom" to the skaters of the Queen City (as Burlington is called). People kept telling her that Burlington needed an indoor skate park. Every Tuesday night, Hannah organized a dinner club. Friends would hit a downtown restaurant, and then head to a local hot spot for dance hall fun. One night, she met a manager of a skate shop from Massachusetts and they started talking; he designed and built skate parks professionally. Drawn together through their similar life interests, they decided to team up on a skateboard business in South Burlington, called Talent Skatepark and Shop.

"We had just signed the lease at Talent and got our loan in 2001, and I was so excited. There was a wallpaper border at the top of a wall, and I wasn't going to open with that ugly wallpaper up there. The ladder was eight feet and it read 'do not stand' on one step but there were two more steps above that. I mean, what are the steps doing there if you can't stand on them? And the top was big enough to stand on. I remember thinking, *I'm going to get so much done while (Dave's) gone.*"

Dave Wood was in Peabody, Massachusetts, building a cement skate park. He was then Hannah's fiancée, now is her husband. "I stood up there, and I had an iron and I was heating the wallpaper and I had a scraper, I was scraping, and something happened." She fell on her left side to the cement floor below.

They brought her to the hospital in the Burlington area, Fletcher Allen Health Care (now the University of Vermont Medical Center). "I had traumatic brain injury on the left side and I had shattered my collarbone," she said. She was put into a medically induced coma for a week and a half. Her brain was swelling badly. They put a shunt in the back of her head and drilled holes to release pressure on the brain caused by swelling.

"I was intubated, and I pulled out the tube twenty-four times and I destroyed my left vocal cord. That's why my voice is a little bit weird." Her mother said she was like a circus contortionist because she would "manipulate, grab, pull" to remove the tube while she was restrained in the bed. "I remember watching *Casper the Friendly Ghost* on television, because my accident was October 17 so all those Halloween things were playing. I had just got engaged, they took all my jewelry, so everyone who came to visit, I would grab their hand, yank off their ring, and stick it on my finger—actually, I don't remember that, it's a story I've been told."

Hannah remembers that she thought the reason she was in the hospital was to care for her roommate, whom she thought was a friend from college, Pat. "It was a woman who looked a lot like this guy, Pat, I bought my first snowboard from. He was a Killington (Vermont) kid, but we knew each other through snowboarding and my crew at the University of Vermont. He had a big, round face and his front teeth were like big (pieces of) Chiclet chewing gum. And the woman in the bed next to me had a big, round face and those teeth. I thought it was Pat and I was there to take care of him."

Hannah was moved to Fanny Allen Campus rehabilitation hospital in Colchester, coincidentally the town in which she grew up (and the same hospital at which I woke up after a couple weeks of post-traumatic amnesia at Dartmouth-Hitchcock Medical Center in Hanover, New Hampshire). Hannah was upset that she was separated from "Pat." It was not Hannah's friend from college years, though Hannah could not be convinced of that. After arguing about her role at the hospital—she still thought she was there as a nurse—David called Hannah's friend Pat in California so Pat could tell her it wasn't him and that he, Pat, was okay.

She was put on antiseizure and antidepression medications, and "probably pain stuff." She stopped taking it. "I didn't want to be on any of it, because I didn't think anything was wrong with me." The doctors wound up putting the meds into soup, and she ate that. She persisted thinking she shouldn't be in the hospital and, like many brain-injury patients, didn't understand her circumstances.

"I had an escape route that I can still see when I go over to Fanny Allen. If I shimmied down the window and there was enough of a ledge, I could edge my way over to the flat roof. And there was a pole, and if I could get to that pole, I was gone. That's when they started locking me in my bed." She was placed in a cage bed, and she said she would kick the bed the whole night, shouting "get me out of here."

When I was in rehab at that hospital, I told Hannah, I snuck over to the computer in the cafeteria one afternoon to furtively check email. Hannah did the same; only she typed "head injuries" in an Internet search and read reports on patients and how their lives were never the same afterward. It was terrifying. "I wish someone had stopped me from that, because everything I read was awful. 'Suicide, taking drugs, life not the same, not the same person'—it was all bad, bad, bad." She began to perseverate, asking her mother over and over, "Am I crazy, am I crazy, am I crazy?" She was terrified of becoming a "crazy person," a vagrant. "Every couple of minutes, I would ask my mother that. I guess I needed her to tell me, no, you're not going to be crazy; you're not going to be a vagrant. I was so afraid."

As every brain is different, cognitive recovery is different for every patient. Hannah began work on speech pathology and cognitive therapy—in other words, recapturing daily life skills.

"One of my biggest struggles after my accident was my voice," she continues. "When you speak the same way for twenty-nine years, you don't realize how much you listen to your own voice—until it sounds different."

When she was released from the hospital, she immediately went back to work at Talent, the skate park she owns and operates. "I think I got out November 23 and we opened Talent December 21, the goal was to get it opened before Christmas." She had voice therapy, and it didn't help. In 2009, she had surgery to repair her vocal cords, which also didn't help. She still sounded as if she was speaking in a whisper. She saw a specialist in Boston, "a top dude" she calls him, and he injected her with Restylane (a substance to aid her vocal cords). Nothing. Her vocal cords were no longer on the same plane, so air wasn't making them vibrate properly. She has decided to live with it. She can't scream, she can't be loud, but she said it's okay. While she was recovering from her brain injury, she said she never had a clear-cut case of aphasia or apraxia. "It was literally the sound of my own voice that bothered me. It was kind of trippy, because I didn't know who was talking, but it was *me*. I didn't recognize the sound of my voice." So she lives with it knowing that "it is a small price to pay for the beauty of life."

She was married to Dave in 2002 and they have two daughters. When their family is relaxing and having fun, she describes experiencing a time vortex that takes her back to when she was a big sister with her younger siblings Sarah and Darah.

"When I'm hanging with my girls, it brings me back to this weird place where they're my younger sisters rather than my children. Not that I want that role, I'm not trying to be that type of parent. But I'll watch them at home, and it's like seeing (my sisters) Sarah and Darah playing. It's freakingly beautiful. That exactly describes how it feels. In raising them, the empathetic side of me is what I focus on with them—sharing the caregiver side. I'm the giver, and I receive. Like, when I donate blood, that's the greatest feeling, it fills me to the brim, I'm high as a kite. My feeling then is: Hey, I just saved three people."

Vermont being a small-population state (second smallest in population, with Wyoming being the smallest in the United States), one of the skateboarders riding at Talent was Kevin Pearce, the snowboarder from Vermont who later had a traumatic brain injury in the half-pipe in Utah while training for the Vancouver Winter Olympics US men's snowboarding team.

Hannah had her accident in 2001, Kevin's crash happened in 2009, and then they connected. After they did, Hannah did a website search on the subject "head injuries" again and this time one of the search results was the Kevin Pearce Fund and the LoveYourBrain outreach campaign.

"All of a sudden, you could Google 'head injuries' and it wasn't 'you're over, you're done' and all that negative stuff. I fell so madly in love with LoveYourBrain because it is what survivors need to thrive! As a head-injury survivor and the owner of a skate park, I probably sell more helmets than anyone in the state of Vermont. LoveYourBrain is perfect and is a foundation I would ultimately like to work for!" she said. "Love is everything."

Stan Perrone, age 60 (as of September 2015)
Hometown: Newtown, CT
Incident: Two years in remission from Stage 4 glioblastoma (a form of brain cancer)

In spring of 2012, after Memorial Day, Stan Perrone decided it was time to hit the pavement, literally—he wanted to jog outside, after months of workouts on an indoor treadmill. Always active, working out five days a week and keeping a journal of his workouts, Stan wanted to kick his physical program into a higher gear. However, he just hadn't felt right for weeks previously. "I didn't feel I was my one-hundred-percent, healthy self." At first, he reasoned he was more out of shape than he had thought. But the feeling persisted. One October day, after going swimming with his grandson, he couldn't seem to get water out of his ear. Then, on a job installing an electrical generator (Stan owns an electrical-contracting company), he came home and told his wife he wanted to eat dinner and go right to bed. As Stan's usually full of energy, she knew something was wrong. He had a fitful night, and in the morning his head pounded. "It's unbearable, it feels like my head's gonna crack," he told his wife. She told him they had to get to the emergency room and they started to get ready. Then she changed her mind and called an ambulance so they could get right in. "The neurosurgeon said that probably saved my life."

An MRI detected a tumor called a glioblastoma in his right temporal lobe. "The problem with brain tumors is that the roots of those cancer cells extend deep into the brain," Karen Perrone said in an article about Stan in the *Newtown Bee*. "Surgeons don't want the surgery to disrupt the healthy brain cells."

The doctor told Stan on the phone they could do surgery the coming Friday, and Stan agreed. "I wanted this out of me, I wanted to do this, I didn't want that thing in there a minute longer than I had to! The doctor said, 'Perfect, that's exactly the attitude I want.'"

The tumor was successfully removed—which Stan had visualized beforehand. His daughter Liz is a nurse practitioner and she told Stan to use positive visual imagery, so he did. "I do that all the time, I do electrical jobs at least once or twice in my head before I even get to the jobsite. She said, 'Well, imagine a positive outcome for the surgery.'"

He said he described his vision or dream to his family, how a young-looking man ("he looked like a Doogie Howser type," Stan said, though Stan hadn't yet met his surgeon) came to his hospital bed "like walking through a cloud" and told him "everything went perfectly." Incredibly, after the surgery, the young-looking Dr. Scott Sanderson came into Stan's room to tell him exactly that.

The golf-ball-size tumor was removed intact and Stan started taking an oral chemotherapy drug, called Temodar, to prevent any remaining cancer cells from growing. He was released from the hospital about a week later and he said he has had no side effects from the surgery and chemotherapy and radiation treatments, except for slight neuropathy in an arm.

Karen and Stan heard about Dr. Keith Block of The Block Center for Integrative Cancer Treatment in Illinois through the Complementary Medicine director at Danbury Hospital (an alternative program in which "the science of medicine meets the art of healing," as the hospital expresses it).

"My wife did some research and she discovered Dr. Block. We met with his entire staff—psychologists, nutritionists. He told us he wants to deal with a strong, healthy patient. He has found that someone who is healthy going in is going to do better with the treatment."

He began an integrative treatment program that included physical, nutritional, and emotional components. Dr. Block learns "what's going on with them uniquely in terms of physical needs, nutritional needs, what's going on with them biochemically. We missed the high touch, because of high tech," and he strives for ways in which patients will respond better to individualized treatments so that outcomes will be better.

Stan had also decided to be positive throughout his treatment, and rejected negative diagnoses such as a doctor telling Karen that glioblastoma is an aggressive cancer that's often terminal in eighteen to twenty-four months. "I surrounded myself with positive information," Stan said. "I feel lucky and blessed, at the same time." Stan had another brain surgery shortly after this first, due to an infection. In October 2014, Stan's brain cancer was two years in remission.

Stan has had strange occurrences during his recovery: "I have this weird ability, when I meditate or pray in the morning before I get out of bed. I sort of let my mind wander, and I can open up these boxes of memories." One April, for instance, he was thinking about calling and wishing his sister, who's nine years younger, a happy birthday—"And

I flashed back to the day my sister was born. I didn't have any recollection of it until that moment. It was like I was watching a video." The temporal lobe is responsible for such functions as visual and auditory perception, as well as memory. Could Stan's super-acute memory be an outcome of his brain cancer? He said he has these sensations from time to time.

He has participated in a program for cancer survivors called Livestrong at a local YMCA, taking step classes, tai chi, strengthening classes, and Zumba. He fondly recalled one experience when they played a song that inspires him, "The Prayer" by Josh Groban and Charlotte Church. After his treatment, he and Karen were part of an advocacy group brought together by the National Brain Tumor Society to help educate legislators about brain tumors and the costs of cancer treatments.

Stan's positive outlook and his physical and mental health clearly have made a difference in his recovery—and now he's helping to spread a positive message for others, as well.

8

WHAT ARE WE DOING TO OURSELVES?

When I graduated college in 1989, I took the headlong plunge into the workforce and that was thrilling, electric—to test my newly acquired academic know-how in the real world and to apply my awakening maturity in the game of adult life. By graduation, I was working part-time at an advertising and public relations agency as an account executive in training; I had started as an intern in my senior year and I had acquitted myself as a dependable (if inexperienced) worker, willing to learn as much as I could about agency marketing and eager to apply the journalism training I had received in college to writing press releases, brochures, and broadcast scripts. I lived in a print world. The agency for which I worked handled mostly print advertising, though we had the Connecticut Lottery account for a while, which was visible business and included radio and television advertising. Television was king, then; advertising on local network TV was expensive, which limited the number of companies who could afford it, which added to the exclusivity of broadcast. Those companies running broadcast were already successful enough to afford it and were reinvesting in marketing and advertising to gain more success. The more common and quotidian business approach—which meant the approach of most businesses—was promotion through print press coverage (newspapers and magazines) augmented and strengthened by print advertising. This was many years before the word *brand* was popularized as a gerund.

I worked hard at applying what I learned in college—print reporting, or back then it was simply "news reporting" as news was transmitted through print newspapers or read from a script on radio or television. I prepared press releases about consumer and business-to-business products (spindle chuckers were a favorite of mine) and served as a liaison to professional news reporters, supplying background information on products and services. I felt I was kind of an adjunct news reporter. I also was a stringer or freelance writer for community newspapers, covering mainly the local sports beat.

There was no consumer Internet, yet, in 1989, so I didn't have "content" to manage through websites or Facebook or Twitter or other social-media outlets. That would come years later. I was able to focus on being an adjunct news reporter and business writer and freelancer. Later, I became a professional editor and writer when I began to manage a magazine-newsletter for New Britain Memorial Hospital, whose clinical focus included traumatic brain injury.

Looking back, I don't remember when email entered my life. It must have been when I took a job as an editor in New York City in 1992. I remember receiving and answered email during that time, but it was rudimentary and certainly not one of the primary means of communication it has become. Ray Tomlinson is generally credited with developing what we now know as email, in 1972. His system gave new meaning to the @ key and helped to popularize the name and place configuration of email addresses.

At that time, 1992, there was no such consumer communication product as a smart phone—the concept would have been science fiction then, as far as I know—and email seemed to be applied internally within organizations, a way to send inner-office notes surreptitiously although I still used handwritten mash notes to reach out to a couple of young women in the New York office.

I was in my twenties when I moved to New York City; I was having a blast working in an office with fellow hedonists, self-possessed and effervescent *bon vivants* whose antics would now be considered self-destructive and at least moderately shameful. We went to long lunches, often. We organized happy hours, often. We had office parties during which we filled plastic trash cans with ice and beer. We did all of this, absolutely, during the workday. We still got our work done, but then again we were a large group of about twenty-five editors, graphic artists, advertising salespeople, print-production people, and support staff. We produced a monthly magazine that averaged about one hundred pages—that is, one hundred *print* pages. There were no ancillary, related electronic-media channels. This magazine had its own circulation staff, routed payables through the corporate accounting office, hired people through the corporate human-resources department—we had corporate support, in addition to the core staff. So we did our individualized jobs and a nine-to-five workday seemed like plenty of time to meet our deadlines each month, twelve months of the year, with an issue each month. We did not have a web department or employees who acted as content creators or information aggregators. At the time, our magazine did not publish a website. No magazine that I knew did then. Social media? Maybe that was the guy who worked in the actual newsstand on the corner of 33rd and Park Avenue?

The nearest we came to social media that I remember was running a national contest in 1994, offering prizes for the best entrants for a new conservation pledge of about thirty words or so that could be recited like the Pledge of Allegiance but in observance of hunting and fishing responsibly and protecting our animal species and natural resources. The magazine's original such pledge was introduced in the 1940s, after World War II, and needed to be updated for the times, the early 1990s. Thousands of people entered their written compositions, which included a fair amount of doggerel; the winner was a policeman from Indiana and he received a new boat, motor, and trailer combo. We read each entry, all of which came through the US mail. My recollection now is that, each year from about 1994 to 2000, email grew in importance and became more critical to staying connected with any constituency, not only to co-workers—but to *everyone*.

After 2000, just about everyone had a handheld, untethered, truly mobile phone; by 2010 or so, everyone seemed to have a smart phone on which email was received and answered. The iPhone was introduced in June 2007. I don't remember that day. But by 2010, I knew I was one of the few who didn't have one and wanted one.

I would not describe myself as a technology adopter of any kind, early or late. Also not a Luddite, I use technology as it relates to my employment. I thought it was cool when I could receive text messages and email on my phone. I thought it was *really* cool when I did get an iPhone in 2011 and began to get it all—email, text messages, and the occasional phone call. Plus, I had the power of a browser in my hand, and could tap into encyclopedic information at any time through a web browser, as long as I had an Internet connection. I didn't realize it then, but I was carrying a pager of sorts—I was always connected.

By gradients, life got faster each year from about 1995 to now and continues to trend that way. More and more was expected of us, professionally. Then it became required of us. Downsizing was common (particularly after the air went out of the economic balloon in 2008) and lean and mean became the new economic mantra. A staff of twenty-five circa 1994 became, through attrition, a staff of fifteen or twelve, yet the deadlines became tighter because now information was required to be immediate if not instantaneous. Real-time was real. Information consumption became continuous, rampant, gluttonous. Fewer people than just a few years previously gathered the information, and did it quickly, and then delivered the information to a forum designed for consumption—mainly, a website. This was true for news, and also for economic reporting and other business information. We needed to know—*now*. There was no patience, and there was no etiquette or equipoise. There was a lot of diplomatic pandering, because you didn't want to piss off anyone. But you had to be faster, faster, faster. The faster you could respond to a request or a question, the better you were, until the next moment when a new need arose. Responding so quickly showed you were highly competent, because you were available right when you were needed!

Because we are always connected—and, right, always needed?—we are always working, really, which means we rarely if ever are free of the pressures and stresses brought on by work. The phrase is 24/7.

"Every day we're assaulted with facts, pseudofacts, news feeds, and jibber-jabber, coming from all directions," wrote Daniel Levitin in *The New York Times* on August 10, 2014. In the same article, he cited a study done in 2011 that reported in a typical day today people take in, or are assaulted by, more information than they would receive in more than 170 newspapers—about five times as much info as we received daily in the mid-1980s. Levitin is a professor at McGill University (Montreal) and author of *The Organized Mind: Thinking Straight in the Age of Information Overload*. Much of what is taking place in our heads is called "executive functioning"—the ability to multitask. The insula appears to be the master switch directing brain activity from immediate-response tasks such as answering email to seeing the new YouTube video, to free-associative pondering or "mind-wandering" as Levitin calls it—in other words, creative thinking that is delightfully non-syllogistic and free-flowing and leads to discoveries thanks to connections of unrelated thoughts in the mind.

Nowadays, the 24/7 approach is how we operate as a culture: We're always connected, always reachable. As a culture, we have been willingly swept up in this roaring wave of connectivity. We've done it as a culture now for more than a decade, and I for one have to ask: Isn't that enough? We've had a front-row seat on the roller coaster through a science-fiction drama of moving faster for the sake of being fast and ever faster. But where are we running to, really? Can we point to tangible progress in our existence of being George Jetson on a treadmill? *Jane, stop this crazy thing!*

When I was writing this part of the book, our house received a lightning strike during an August thunderstorm. The electrical discharge surged through power wires and, even though the modem was plugged into a circuit-breaker power strip, our family's Internet was fried, coming to an end with an audible *snap*. Practicing accept-ance, I quelled my stress and continued with a regular life for three days without Internet connectivity. Caught in a web of connected-ness throughout my professional life, I had to adjust to being discon-nected for a couple of weekdays, and I felt faintly irresponsible about it. All the publishing projects with which I was involved continued apace; I visited the local library to use their Internet connection, I survived. This was a good test; I would not have always reacted with a controlled and measured response; prior to my brain injury, my stress would have reached zenith levels, I know—I would have lost my mind over this.

I heard scientist Jon Kabat-Zinn (on YouTube, of course) refer to modern people as "human doings, rather than human beings." He pointed out in his talk on University of California TV, promoting his book *Coming to Our Senses*, that we won't get all our daily tasks done because there is no end to the tasks. There are always more.

Kabat-Zinn was a pioneer of Mindfulness Based Stress Reduction (MBSR) at the Stress Reduction Clinic at the University of Massachusetts Medical School. He received his PhD in molecular biology from Massachusetts Institute of Technology. He became involved with yoga and Buddhist teachings and this led him to mind-fulness as a discipline and practice, which he introduced clinically. As a scientist, he has been a distinguished and elegant advocate for integrating Buddhist teachings into Western medicine. His book *The Mind's Own Physician: A Scientific Dialogue with the Dalai Lama on the Healing Power of Meditation*, which he coedited with Richard Davidson of University of Wisconsin-Madison, came out of the Mind and Life Institute Dialogue with the Dalai Lama in 2005. The Institute was founded in 1987 with the Dalai Lama and scientists exploring syner-gies between science, contemplative traditions, and philosophy, the goal of which was "to promote well-being on the planet." It's been an effort to investigate how we can better manage our minds and do good work with our brains. From the organization's website, www.mindandlife.org:

For the past thirty years, the Mind and Life Institute has pioneered the field of contemplative science. In pairing the oldest wisdom traditions with cutting-edge scientific research, contemplative science uncovers groundbreaking and holistic insights into the human mind and condition. These insights represent some of the most important breakthroughs of our time. Mind and Life's work operates in an array of rigorous fields—neuroscience, psychology, education, medicine, ethics, religion, the humanities—and is always guided by the Institute's larger mandate to alleviate suffering, cultivate kindness and compassion, and advance human flourishing.

This investigation introduces ideas of great consequence to our culture. We might enable ourselves to escape what the poet William Blake called "mind-forg'd manacles" or mind-created suffering that includes stress and anxiety. So often, these seem beyond our control. Self-centered craving, greed, hatred, delusion, debasement, resentment, ignoble thinking or intent, arrogance, jealousy, obsessive desire, negativity—these are bred from *dukkha* or the Buddhist word for dissatisfaction or an unquiet mind. In the aforementioned book, Ajahn Amaro, one of the moderators, wrote that meditation is a pathway to "focus the attention and capacity to investigate, explore, and contemplate the nature of experience itself."

Recently, I saw a bumper sticker that read MY KARMA RAN OVER MY DOGMA. As a dog-lover, I thought that was harsh—but funny, in the fleeting way bumper stickers are. But I don't feel thinking about *dukkha* is dogmatic, rather it's practical. It's humanistic. Getting to know ourselves is a natural process, or should be.

Mindfulness meditation is a means of turning inward with self-examination, or curious observation. The latter part is beautiful, to me: To be curious about oneself and to contemplate the decisions of our own brain. To better grasp why we do the things we do and to observe ourselves and consider our own brain in operation. If you focus your thoughts hard enough, can you imagine the synapses connecting? Can you feel your own energy, expressed as thought, and be courageous enough to detach from the thoughts and simply to observe them in action? Not to act on any, necessarily, but simply to observe?

Matthieu Ricard is quoted as saying in *The Mind's Own Physician:* "meditation means familiarity with qualities that we have the potential to enhance, like unconditional compassion, openness to others, and inner peace." It helps us to achieve "familiarization with the very way the mind works." This is the same Ricard, the Buddhist monk from Nepal, who was a study subject in Richard Davidson's brain monitoring at University of Wisconsin-Madison and exhibited impressively powerful gamma-wave brain readings while practicing loving-compassion meditation.

Meditation may be an answer for us and allow us to step off the George Jetson treadmill we've allowed ourselves to be tethered to, perhaps unwittingly and unknowingly. That's what happens when we sacrifice awareness—we lose control over ourselves, literally. Our cognitive pathways become jangled, aberrant, overloaded.

Our very scientific name *Homo sapiens sapiens* means "species that knows and knows that he knows"—sentient and conscious. Too often, we want to forget that we know because answering that email is so immediately more important than isolated thoughts; and feeling connected is more immediately gratifying than being all alone. I understand that our humanity craves contact and we feel gratified by the importance of being needed and giving help. But do we have to Tweet to our followers that we just had a funny thought? Or do we really have to show our Instagram audience our latest fun (for whom?) or silly photo? Why report out in this way?

Why not embrace *being* and be in the moment of *now.*

Much mindfulness and Buddhist teaching emphasizes the inner power we have—for example, the Mind and Life Institute discusses alleviating suffering through attention, emotional balance, kindness, compassion, confidence, and happiness. Becoming more directly in touch with our inner power might be a start of a re-entry plan to life. I don't recommend falling on your head as a way to clear the gunk from the folds of your brain. I don't know—nor do neurologists—what causes the gunk (is it the protein tau?) to accumulate amid the folds of our brains, the sulci and gyri, probably resulting in all of that surface area of tissue being compromised. In this way, synapses won't fire, brain pathways or modules or modalities won't wire together, and plasticity no longer occurs. Of course, the gunk may be figurative and it's merely our choice to short-circuit our own thinking.

My father, in his mid–seventies, has Alzheimer's and was diagnosed with it in 2005. His memory is still with him, both long-term and short-term. He has no apparent dementia. He is forgetful and doesn't seem to process thoughts, ideas, and responses with alacrity. My mother, his wife of more than five decades who knows him better than anyone, thinks he may have also suffered a stroke ten years ago. He complained to her of not feeling well when he came in from fishing in South Florida, he lay down, and he napped. He never returned to being the man I've known my entire life. Of course, I'm concerned about the genetic material I'm carrying. Now that I'm aware of my brain and understand the processes at work up there, I want to keep the lights fully on, as long as possible.

My grandmother on my father's side died deeply enveloped in dementia. She was a tough lady, raised eight children by herself as my paternal grandfather did not help (so I've been told, he died before I was born), since he was too distracted by alcohol. There was enough of an age difference among the children (my father and aunts and uncles) that the oldest sibling cared for the youngest, but that's not the same as having a parent attentive to every whim, cry, and need. My father was an introverted man for most of his adult life, constantly reminding his three young children that we were a private family and did not discuss family matters publicly. He was adamant about privacy, perhaps because he grew up communally with his brothers and sisters. So I became a writer and have a deep passion and appreciation for learning and sharing stories. That feels satisfying.

Both my parents were teachers and have an inveterate aptitude for and true tropism toward sharing knowledge (with combined teaching experience of more than fifty years) and were pleased watching their children develop—while also being compassionate disciplinarians and putting the fear of reprisal into us if they saw us not trying.

My older brother (by less than two years) and my younger sister (by about three years) and I did work hard, learned to creatively cut corners where and when we could, learned to value the importance of interpersonal skills, and have so far achieved stable lives with nuclear and extended families showing love and care. We learned love and care, first, and now we dwell in love and care.

I've abided by love and care, compassion and empathy, throughout my life, though also have been hampered by restlessness and imaginative yearnings that extend the scope of my mind in distracted extrapolation. I think too much. Which leads me back to being mindful of the internal monologue inside me that became a mind-forged, incessant, self-contemptuous trap. I don't say that with hostility directed toward myself or with cloying, psychosomatic judgment. I simply have a measure of before August 14, 2012, and after. The interior monologue was present inside me and I never bothered to be curious about it and really examine and observe my own thoughts. I find that change exciting now, and although I have bouts of self-criticism and cynicism, I recognize the meaning I wear around my neck and have for fifteen years: The Divine Abidings, the "four immeasurables" of loving-kindness (or love), compassion, joy, and equanimity. When I woke up from my amnesia, I eventually became aware that the necklace I'd worn was missing, as the emergency crew or doctors had removed it. It is a piece of jewelry that inspired me to reproduce crude facsimiles of the Sanskrit symbols for *Maitri, Karuna, Mudita, Upeksha* on my shower wall, where I could be alone with the words each morning and allow some of the meaning to wash over me.

That was years before my accident, when I was searching for some meaning beyond the Catholic faith in which I was raised. Many aspects of Catholicism I find beautiful—apart from the Sunday mass itself, which is usually dire and repetitive and rote and contains too much reflection on guilt and sorrow, for me. To the contrary, the sacred writing of the Upanishads contains beauty. For many years in my twenties, I was enamored with the Isa Upanishad and used as a personal mantra the verse "Behold the universe in the glory of God: and all that lives and moves on earth. Leaving the transient, find joy in the Eternal: set not your heart on another's possession."

I repeated this before teeing off on a golf course, while sitting on the subway, before going to bed, casting a fly into a New York City reservoir, while sitting on a barstool in the White Horse Tavern or 119 Bar or Molly's Shebeen. The words fortified me. The language pacified me. I felt better, saying this phrase. Reading brought me similar ease—though often I also read for instruction on writing.

I mention this to document that beauty had an intellectual attraction for me and so too I was striving to sharpen the meaning of the beauty of life transmitted through my thoughts. I can't lay claim to any particular strain of enlightenment, but as a writer I did yearn (and still do) to know more about how lives are lived and why.

This was a connection to the implicit knowledge gained through emotion, the guiding direction of my hippocampus, perhaps, the automatic unconsciousness heightening my awareness of the collective of humanity. I feel parallel plasticity enabled my brain to cognitively probe into understanding an awareness of humanity and an understanding of selfhood. I don't think I was, or am, too full of shit about that.

I was given a tremendously valuable gift when I was a boy. My father took me fishing. We moved to a lakeshore when I was nine and water became a foundational element in my life. The amygdala delivered my consciousness to water during the weeks when I was not conscious in the hospital—these are the escapist dreams I remember.

I have a memory after my fall of being on a lake in what seemed to be the Adirondack Mountains, which I had visited with my family as a child. We stayed at Sabattis, a lake and campground named for Mitchell Sabattis. Mitchell Sabattis was an Abenaki Native American and famous Adirondack guide, the son of an Adirondack pioneer, and died in the early 1900s in Long Lake, New York. "In the woods he saw and heard and reasoned with a refinement that was uncanny," Alfred L. Donaldson recalled in his book *A History of the Adirondacks*. Sabattis killed his addiction—alcohol—and went on to local fame as a preacher and sportsman. A wide passage of Adirondack land was named in his honor, in which access for all was guaranteed. Now, Camp Sabattis is a Boy Scout retreat.

This memory appeared when I was in the hospital and my brain was either conflicted about where I was or confused about *who* I was—so the protective part of the brain at that time, the amygdala, directed me to a familiar and safe element—water—and the beautiful surrounding environs of a rural shoreline, possibly in the Adirondacks. It was vivid and extremely peaceful, restful, safe. The sun was setting over the small lake in front of me, suspended just over the treetops. There was an ease in the air, as I had experienced for many years at dusk on the lake on which I grew up in Central New York. I can now see the scene and I can believe that my brain was preparing me—for death, perhaps? If this was the last experience I ever had . . . maybe it was so I could recall it with pleasure in the next wherever?

Or was this a precursor to embarking upon a different life, a cosmic foreshadowing of the years to come? I also remember fishing with my friend Harry in the Adirondacks and watching him cast a fly rod; in my dreamscape, I gently offered a suggestion to him *not* to brake the casting wrist until the very end of the presentation cast, so as to force the artificial fly to land on the water's surface meniscus with a slight shudder or plop, which can attract the attention of fish underneath and create an irresistible image in their upward-looking search image for food. I remember the sensation of feeling completely secure, like the nighttime sound of bullfrogs from the lake I heard as a child always brought a sense of ease and security.

After I woke up and came to my senses, or my senses once again became functional I continued to have recurrent theme dreams of this nature, which I now remember, but only a few as they must have dissipated as my recovery continued to become active and my awareness heightened. I feel certain now this was an act of the amygdala, infusing reassurance into the general pool of memory in my brain. Scattered memories were leaking into my consciousness. It helped me recapture who I was when I woke up.

Since I've been awake now for less than two years as I write this, I want to preserve this feeling I possess about life. I've learned that the only life we have is the now. Try as we might, we can't control our past or shape our future. Similarly, we can learn from past experience and by not repeating undesirable behaviors and actions, we can save ourselves anguish and pain. We grow as we apply what we learn. It's simple in theory, more challenging in practice.

I feel much more attuned to a 4/4 time signature, in this way. I had gone through an adolescent phase with my life tempo pulsing to 2/4 time and the associated identity of punk rock and nihilism and in my early adult years that did remain as an echo in my brain, and contributed to the internal metronome of time signature that set a fractious, herky-jerky internal tempo for me, particularly in times of stress and anguish.

Instead, the 4/4 time that's settled in me today is more measured and relaxed and is a tempo that leads to deliberate progress, which is the vital in vitality. This feeling and notion of moving forward in a measured time signature, I feel, leads to emotional progress and a willfulness to work on improving my behavior, progressively, without judgment.

Fishing taught me regulation. Fishing taught me an incredible amount about patience—you can't will a wild animal to eat, you have to wait, try other approaches and techniques—but the sport also taught me about keeping focus in the now. Here's a mental exercise: Imagine a weightless facsimile of an insect tied to a nearly invisible strand of extruded plastic, about as sheer as a material can be and still hold a knot of the material folded over itself and have the molecular strength to support the knot clinching a metal loop at the head of the fly. The fake insect is a fishing fly, tied to a tippet, which is tied to a slightly heavier piece of extruded plastic (monofilament), which is attached to a plastic-coated line called a fly line because its purpose is to cast the weightless fake fly. Once that casting motion impels enough energy to overcome inertia, and the fake bug is delivered to the water, the tippet must be strong enough to hold its clinch on the metal loop so that when an aquatic organism mistakes the fake fly for a real insect and gulps it, the connection will extend almost immediately through the sections of line and to a graphite rod held by an angler. The fish and the angler are now connected by several sections of line knotted together, hinging on a loop around metal at the end of the fake fly, which holds the fish on the point of an extremely thin metal hook. Shock absorption is designed into the flexible properties of the wire or thin-metal hook and the give and flex of the extruded plastic line and the plastic-coated, braided-core fly line, all further cushioned by the flex in the nine-foot, tapered graphite (or bamboo or fiberglass) rod, and regulated by a click-and-pawl or disc-controlled mechanism called a drag meting out line incrementally when pulled by the fish. Because of the tenuous relationship of the parts, all will fail if any one part fails. The margin is slight and all is fraught through with possible dissolution. Success starts when the fish eats your fake insect and culminates when the angler brings the wild aquatic creature to hand, only to release it back into the wild or to kill it. Your encounter with the power of the fish's life force is fleeting, either way.

This experience is meditation. It is fluid, while under way, and requires your complete attention. You're aware of the constants of beauty all around you, whether wading in a stream like the Firehole in Yellowstone National Park and casting deliberately for cutthroat trout and conducting the ballet of constantly mending fly line upstream; or if you're standing on a platform at the bow of a boat in the Florida Keys casting heavier fly tackle and larger flies for *Megalops atlanticus* or tarpon, the smell of musty mangroves and sulfurous gas in the breeze. Meditation also occurs when creating the flies you'll be casting for these fish, sitting at a desk far from the water and wrapping thread around the stems of chicken feathers or elk hair and around the thin hook. The focus of wrapping a feather in a spiral around the hook shank is a technique called palmering a hackle, and the barbules of the feather open up to create the impression of legs and antennae and buggy-looking life. This is meditation, focus, being in the now.

In Montana, I was sitting in an inflatable boat—a raft—positioned in the bow, casting across my body and forcing down the grasshopper-imitating fly with a plop on the water's surface. I knew I was in a beautiful place, but my focus was intent on the mechanics of moving my right forearm back toward my shoulder, and pushing it forward. When the fly landed on the water, after a five-one-thousand count as the fly drifted downstream, I flicked it back over my head and forced it down again—and the water erupted when the fly landed. A huge trout rolled after eating the fly, and I yanked up with the rod, breaking the sheer tippet while the water receded after the eruption, with a hiss. We were floating down the Smith River in Montana and drifting past a rock cliff against which the river flowed. Big trout positioned themselves underwater against the cliff, waiting for insects to fall to the water's surface, at which point they would engulf the bugs. Meditation and therapy.

As we floated the river, my oarsman Bill Yellowtail and I talked about life. Bill was raised on his family's ranch, on the Crow Reservation in Montana and served as a Montana state senator. He radiated spirituality, and while I snored away a night after drinking Scotch by the campfire he slept in a sleeping bag outside, no tent over his head. We floated and fished the river all day, beached the boats and made camp for dinner and slept soundly each night. This was one of the great experiences of my life, filled with meditation, as I think back on it now. Waking each morning with full attention on considering the insects on which the trout might be feeding, and adjusting the day's fly box to include Sofa Pillows (large mayfly imitations) or yellow, rubber-legged and weighted Wooly Buggers (leech imitations). Bill and I stopped and hiked up a streamside trail to the Indian pictographs on cave walls, ancient rock art, finger lines and hand impressions, and smears and animal forms.

This is a form of meditation that preserves one's sanity in a world that drives us to ever more irrational behavior. Being disconnected is a good strategy and the truest way I've found in my life to accomplish relief from the insidious, mind-dominating tremors of modern life . . . is fly fishing. You can study lots of wonderful minutiae like the bio forms of insects and minnows and invertebrates and fish rise forms (the manner in which trout eat) and how to create imitations of foodstuff of trout and bonefish and tarpon and then actually make the imitations (knitting for men, a friend calls tying flies), all of which force you to slow down and consider your actions. Let's not neglect the mechanics of fly casting, and where to hold your dominant arm and how you position your body to be efficient and effective. Then look around and admire the beauty—the sport takes us to some awfully incredible places. (As does wingshooting, with a tinge of sadness at the denouement of killing a gamebird.)

I think of standing thigh-deep in saltwater on the south shore of Montauk Point, New York. Striped bass splash and thrash as a sizable school of fish ambushed bay anchovies (a type of minnow) and I was furiously casting my fly rod to deliver a fly I had made called a Clouser Minnow into the seething biomass of fish and bait. The fly, weighted with lead eyes so a bit easier to cast than an unweighted fly and sinking immediately once hitting the water, landed in the foamy wave wash, and I tugged on my fly line to give the fly some movement that approximated life. A fish pulled back and I tugged the line to hook a migratory ocean fish on the fly I had tied a few nights before sitting at my desk in Vermont. I slipped on seaweed and nearly fell and when I looked down into the water, I saw the red-brown shell of a lobster tumbling through the longshore current. I held my fly rod aloft with my right arm as the fish's twists and turns produced thumps of the line against the rod, and I crouched and pinched the lobster by its shell and picked it up with my left hand so I could gauge its size, about a pound. The migratory striped bass, passing through the waters off Montauk Point on their way south from Stellwagon Bank or Martha's Vineyard and returning to their home water (and probably birthwaters) in Chesapeake Bay in instinctual response to a drive for food or triggered by water temperature or moon phase (or both), was attached to my line, and resisted my nine-foot fly rod and the reel's drag, while I held a lobster in the air and laughed a hearty guffaw.

I remember saying my Isa Upanishad prayer, "Behold the universe in the glory of God . . ." and feeling the surge of the surf and the pull of the water's retreat. Surely, there was no importance here, a lone angler standing in the shallows of the Atlantic Ocean, holding a short lobster in one hand and with the other trying to control a traveling fish desperate to escape death (though I would and did release the fish)—nothing important, except the absolute significance of that moment as life converged and somehow I was part of the nexus.

9

THE EMOTIONAL BRAIN

I write this on the day before the two-year anniversary of my climbing the ladder and plummeting to Earth—August 14, 2012, was the day or (most probably) afternoon when my fall occurred. My wife and I recently ordered a family gift that was delivered a day ago (again, as I write this)—a new Coleman tent, as my son and I often camp in our backyard at a fire pit I built with stones repurposed from an old fieldstone wall that lines our property from the times when all the land on our ridge was working farm, so the trees were all cleared (as was about 80 percent of the state of Vermont) and boundaries and property lines were marked by stones removed from the cleared fields. My son and I opened the shipping box and he announced, "Dada, we're camping tonight!" in the bossy and declarative manner of a six-year-old. So it was decided. I would spend the night about a hundred yards from where I came to rest on August 14, 2012, at the base of a maple tree.

We erected the tent in our usual spot, where our hilly lawn slopes out under two apple trees, adjacent to the fire pit. It's a sizable tent, as the difference in floor to ceiling clearance between a twenty-year-old four-person tent (our previous model) and a modern six-person tent is considerable. The higher domed roof is the biggest difference between the two, allowing me and my wife, both of us taller than six feet, to stand up inside.

We had dinner and then I started the campfire, and readied the site. My wife read to my son and they bedded down in the tent, a nap for my wife and sleepy time for my son, and I finished a work project inside at my desk (the desk from which I remember seeing the black cat in the tree, on August 14). I moved outside after darkness fell, sitting for a while in front of the fire to read. My wife awoke and went inside the house to sleep in our bed. I felt a gravity emanating from the maple tree about a hundred yards from where I sat, now bathed in moonlight from a Grain Moon four nights before and waning now to gibbous, brilliant in the absolutely clear sky. After reading for about an hour, I closed the book and waded through the moonlight to the base of the maple.

A barred owl was calling aggressively west across the road, dueling with another barred before the shrill call of a great horned owl pierced the night. I lay down on the lawn to study my breath and empty my thoughts, regarding the branches and leaves in silhouette. I recited the first stanza of the Isa Upanishad, a couple of times. I relaxed my body and tried to remember—what happened that day? Did I step onto a branch and lose my balance, or did I try to jump from ladder to limb? Was I reaching outward and simply slipped and fell? Nothing. I concentrated and then my mind began to create histories and scenarios. I was standing on a branch coaxing the cat, and then threatening her. I was climbing the tree, as I'm sure the cat was higher than I was looking right then. Or was it? I don't know. I never will. What happened that day was commonplace, really; what's happened afterward is the discovering of the blessing of this life—my "wild and precious life," now actual. As I lay on the lawn, supine, I had observed the anniversary I felt in the proper fashion, communing with the maple tree that had held me before my plunge earthward, continuing into a brief period of nothingness while my brain took a breather and reordered.

I walked back to my lawn chair at the fire, studying the fire and watching the flames hop and jump, the sparks rising and flittering and briefly orbiting the fire pit like caddisflies, and then disappearing as the individual sparking embers dimmed and extinguished. The flash and splash of the firelight lit the vinyl tent shell to my right, the hum and hiss of the fire mingling with the light snore and sleep groan of my son inside.

The fire triggered a memory—which in itself is incredible, that I can summon memories or have them float up in my consciousness arbitrarily, a seemingly rote occurrence for which I am so grateful and that I do not for an instant take for granted. In fact, I continue to have a true feeling of blessedness for my cognition, now that I've learned a little about how we function. The triggered memory was of a horse-pack trip in the early 1990s to the Wind River Range of Wyoming, sitting with others on the trip (a media outing arranged by a compass manufacturer) encircling a campfire, the firelight outlining each member sitting in the group of six or eight. One of the trip directors asked each of us to talk about what we were thankful for, and what we'd ask for if we could talk with our creator. He asked us to share. We were on a Native American Reservation and had Shoshone and Arapaho guides leading us and one of the guides, I remember his name as Big Jim, said, "I'd ask the man, 'What's it all about? This life, I mean, what it's all about?'" This seemed an ecumenical moment, as I thought back the twenty-something years.

Two years had passed since I lay on the lawn—unconscious, inert, in the scrub at the base of the tree, unaware but at least still alive. Emerging into a new consciousness, weeks and months later.

As I watched the fire, I thought about my nucleus accumbens, a part of my brain responsible for capturing and nurturing pleasure responses. I was thinking of it courtesy of my insula, which gives me perception and makes me aware of and is possibly attuned to my body and physical state, science thinks.

After my injury, in rehab, a therapist had explained to me a possible outcome common among the brain injured called perseveration, the speech center (Broca's area) repeating the same thought or expression over and over, skipping like a stereo needle in the microgroove of a vinyl LP, the patient thinking and then saying the same word or phrase repeatedly. I was terrified of this happening to me. I thought about it: How would I know this was happening? Was I self-aware enough to know? If I knew I was doing it, I would stop doing it, right? So it would be happening outside of memory? It was an existential puzzle, straining my ability to reason that early in my recovery. Then I would reassure myself that if I could reason, I must have self-awareness and therefore would not perseverate.

Ah (I later learned), the insula was likely coming to my aid. Perceptions were intact and my emotional experience also seemed moderated, thanks to my still-functioning prefrontal cortex. I was not perseverating. I didn't. I had injured my left frontal lobe—but not enough to do permanent, catastrophic injury. I was slower, that much I knew. I couldn't react immediately to any stimulus—a question, anything I read, or even processing a passive statement heard on TV. In that example, I would hear the statement and the auditory information would proceed through a processing cycle for a few seconds before I formed a responding thought. I took it in and needed a couple beats before an answer or reaction took shape. This was true of tactile impulses felt through my fingers, too, I noticed. I would slowly go ahead with physical reactions—watching a mosquito on my left arm for a second before understanding that I should squash it and then moving my right arm to squash—but I was more tentative and hesitant with decisions.

Sometimes, I didn't commit immediately because I wanted to rehearse an answer in my head *first* before I delivered it for real—my mind became an internal fact-checker. Certainly this was my protective ego at work—I didn't want to appear deficient so I would pause to reflect before answering. But I'm not sure there was anything I could do about these slower reactions. I'm more deliberate, and I think my way through a thought or action—very different from being on autopilot and acting reflexively, the way I lived life before my injury.

I still am slower with my responses—slower in my cognitive *processing,* really—two years later. My thoughts filter through my mind a bit more labored than before my fall, I need a couple of moments—mere seconds, but pauses nonetheless—to compose a sensible answer to a question, no matter how simple or for that matter how conversationally complex. I am rarely able to be on autopilot. I am in the moment, because I have to be. I don't always rehearse in those seconds, but sometimes I do. I work in my mind at enunciation, most of all. I find myself overemphasizing diction to be as precise as I can with the sound I'm trying to make while vocalizing a word. I surprise myself with my ability to say multisyllabic words like *quintessentially,* but then slur a simple word like *sleep* making it *seep.* My inner fact-checker is also my inner Henry Higgins/Rex Harrison in *My Fair Lady.* (I should also mention—my inner fact-checker is also much gentler than my inner voice or interior monologue used to be.)

I think now—*Okay, I'm nearing fifty so this is going to happen, I'm going to get slower.* Maybe my injury exacerbated or accelerated the onset of this condition but it's pretty natural all the same, this slowness, or at least understandable to others as they see the gray in my beard and acknowledge that I'm middle-aged. Broca's area, where speech is produced, is working okay. After my injury, the doctors were concerned that Wernicke's area, and even more so Broca's area, could be at risk of direct injury due to my left frontal impact. Wernicke's seems proficient, but there is a nagging delay between the formation of words (including my internal knowledge of their meanings) and the muscle contractions that allow me to form and voice the words. This is not only a spoken effect. I've experimented with writing the words, rather than saying them. No better, still a delay. Which is why I say, it seems to be the time of my processing that's changed. I used to consider myself a quick and vivid thinker—quick with a quip, a joke, a comeback. That was my former self-identity. I'm no longer that way. And to that, I say: so what?

Knowing the parts of the brain responsible for certain functions is relatively new to me—two years new, in fact. Remarkable—how could I have gone for so long without a burning curiosity about my brain function and behavior and the reasons for doing what I do, I ask myself now. For forty-three years, I was making choices and decisions, and thinking intensely about expressing my thoughts, opinions, and desires. But I was on autopilot, too distracted by worries of past events and concerns about the future to appreciate being in the present now.

As I sat staring into the fire on August 14, a verse formed in my mind . . . it was Rabindranath Tagore:

In a wordless, lightless, great emptiness, Four-faced Brahma broods.

This came to me from the recesses of memory, triggered perhaps by watching the fire in the dark. It was Rabindranath Tagore, the Bengali poet, and the poem is "Brahma, Vishnu, Shiva," which I read in his collected works many years before my head injury. I learned of Tagore from studying William Butler Yeats, who admired Tagore and helped with translations of his work from Bengali to English. The two were friends for nearly forty years, history tells us. Contemporaries, both were awarded Nobel Prizes for their work, Tagore ten years before Yeats.

I'm moved by memories of verse from Yeats, "Turning and turning in the widening gyre" and my time in the void of no memory.

I went to an isle in the water, I know that, during my mostly dark incapacitation after my fall. I know nothing from that time, nearly a month, yet I remember going to an island in the water at some point after my injury. I can still see the leaves on the trees, and the trees on the shore, and the bushy beard or sweet flag growing thick along the shore. I remember the unfurling of a fly line being cast by my friend Harry. I smile in appreciation of having this capacity of memory still, that my neurotransmitters were firing and the inner sea of connectivity in my head had a live current when my consciousness was otherwise dark. My brain took me to a safe place—was it my amygdala orchestrating an escape? Yes, I feel it was.

I'm abuzz with intellectual excitement—Christmas for my brain!—
to read the new book by Haruki Murakami after devouring the enco-
mium on him by none other than the rocker Patti Smith in *The New
York Times* Sunday *Book Review* on August 10, 2014. So much of what
I love about literature is contained in that review! Who decided Patti
Smith should be the one to write about Murakami's work? Making
me part of the attentive audience being told to "keep living because
only by living can you see what happens next." I dive into Murakami
on the Kindle.

Another fear besides the onset of perseveration entered my thoughts
during recovery—resulting from unsteady mental orientation, no
doubt, it cropped up fleetingly until a therapist gave me a direct warning: Depression can settle into the recovering mind.

An article in the Brain Injury Association of America's journal
The Challenge! reported a direct linkage of traumatic brain injury and
depression, though whether that results from inflammation of the
brain is unclear. Certainly, the awareness of one's changed abilities and
deficiencies, whether short- or long-term, result in at least morose if
not depressed thoughts. The article also mentions that TBI survivors
"often demonstrate disinhibition, or impulsive behavior, which may
include reacting suddenly to emotions without first considering the
consequences of behavior."

Impulse control is an issue for TBI survivors. Further, the rigors
of recovery are exacerbated by the sense of loss: loss of oneself or the
sense of self and the unreliability of aptitude and mental abilities here-
tofore taken for granted before the injury or insult, due to changes
in baseline cognitive functions, the therapist I was seeing told me.
Depression is a common outcome for TBI patients, apparently once
you realize you're not the same.

I reflected on this: We know we're not the same in many ways or
even every way, but we want to prove we are no different than we
were. We've got a big something to prove. This is as tough as it gets—
it's the brain we're talking about!

My friend Sue Shirland, the equestrian who had a brain and spinal injury in 1990, told me about her mental struggles. "I didn't like myself. My sense of self was very diminished. I couldn't talk right, I couldn't ride right. I was so frustrated that my body wouldn't do what it was supposed to do," she said. "I didn't like living in this new environment. I didn't think I was very worthy, why would anyone want to be around me?"

In my short time talking with her, I would describe Sue as lively and introspective. But when you don't recognize your core self and you feel your essence is different, I understand so well how you can feel lost and become depressed. "I was just incompetent. I couldn't do anything right. Sue told me." Her family doctor was a friend and she went to see him professionally. "Our family physician (in Vermont) is Allan Ramsay. We're good friends, but when you go to see him in his office, he's the doctor. I went to see him in May or June after my spinal surgery. He asked me, 'Have you thought about suicide?' I said yes. And he asked, 'How you gonna do it?' And I told him I hadn't figured that out yet. I didn't know how, but it had to be something that didn't upset Larry (Sue's husband). It couldn't be gross. [The doctor] put me on some medication and it helped."

The author and psychologist Kay Jamison, in her memoir *An Unquiet Mind*, wrote:

"I long ago abandoned the notion of a life without storms, or a world without dry and killing seasons. Life is too complicated, too constantly changing, to be anything but what it is." Jamison writes that the difficulties remind us that we're alive. That puts me in mind of Beckett and *Waiting for Godot* . . . eh, Didi?

I think now and recognize an echo of uncertainty I had while stretched on my hospital bed and later shuffling to the bathroom or to the day's therapy appointments. There were tremors of disquiet within me, a sense that something had changed and was different. This happened days after the nurse congratulated me for waking up, as my amnesia lifted. Through the previous weeks, I didn't recognize myself when I stared into a mirror, which I often did for hours, I've been told, trying to parse how I knew this some-how familiar face. Perhaps I did that clinically, unemotionally, so it caused no internal distress or mental strife in that lost soul who was me? My brother, who was with me days after my injury, told me I stared in the mirror and stroked my beard—until I shaved it off with a Norelco electric razor my mother-in-law bought for me. Maybe that was to reveal the skin underneath and therefore have a better way to recognize the clean-shaven man? My fusiform gyrus kept coming up empty, with no recognition and no answers. This is also when I was restrained in my bed and considered a flight risk. Courtesy of the fight-or-flight amygdala, the impulse was to get the hell out of this situation.

Which makes me wonder, 150 years ago if I had been struck in the frontal lobe by a Minie Ball at Appomattox and survived, how would I have ever recovered? Would I have been considered insane or, worse, possessed by evil (worse than ergot poisoning)? In any case, recovery would likely have been out of the question, as infection probably would have ended my tumult and my life.

Throughout my recovery, I did not spiral into depression. But the more I felt the traction of recovery, the more the pinch of depres-sive thoughts came, thanks again to the amygdala and its partners the hippocampus and thalamus. I knew something about me was differ-ent. In the book *Head Cases: Stories of Brain Injury and Its Aftermath*, by Michael Paul Mason, one head-injury survivor is quoted as say-ing, "I'm not me anymore, but I'm still me." I felt that. There was a specter looming just outside my awareness that was cloaked in panic and fear.

Kay Jamison wrote in *An Unquiet Mind* that "Depression is flat, hollow, and unendurable. It is also tiresome." I can appreciate this. I describe my experience following my traumatic brain injury as filled with bouts of confusion, but thankfully not despair.

I know I'm lucky that depressive thoughts did not root in my brain. Instead, I felt a return to my core, and delighted in a sense of recon-nectedness to life. (I'll share more about that in the next chapter on recovery.) I was recharged and emotionally resolute and determined. That was my experience—but I have to caution that depression is a real risk after a brain injury. Our sense of self is so often precarious and constantly changing and mutable. When it is altered because of changes in cognitive function—when we truly lose ourselves—the result to the injured can be catastrophic and the thinking can become terminal.

I started conversational therapy shortly after I was released from the hospital and I have to think sharing my doubts and vulnerabilities neutralized them and certainly lessened their importance in my mind. My internal monologue, to this day, has not returned to its previous controlling, discursive, distracting degree nor does it have anywhere near the internal vocal power as before my head injury. Today, my thoughts are still a constant, always with me, just not a constant badgering or nattering. I'm more at peace—and I love life.

10

DEEPER INTO RECOVERY

Recently, I read "Brain injuries cannot be managed any more than a thunderstorm can be managed," in *Head Cases: Stories of Brain Injury and Its Aftermath* by Michael Paul Mason, a fascinating collection of brain-injury recovery stories, ranging from collision injuries— including a gripping story about old-school snowboarder Cheyenne Emerick's crash while snowboarding in Utah—to medical conditions and genetic manifestations. Brain-injury recovery cannot be managed, no. It takes time and, just as with all that's meaningful and valuable in life, hard work, repetition, and practice. Repeatedly realizing our true human value, it seems to me.

How to prioritize? As I was told by survivor Sue Shirland: "I just picked something and I just worked at it until I got it," she said. "That's something you do in dressage, you prioritize. You work on things, it's a progression. Analyze and prioritize."

I'll share more about what I faced when my amnesia lifted. When my recovery began, I started with establishing the simple facts of the day, and I made them real by having them written down—my room number, why I was in the hospital and where that was, what had happened, the date, the day of the month. I had difficulty writing, due to the cast on my right arm, so the lead therapist wrote out that information for me in my wide-ruled composition notebook, my memory aid. I was placed (I learned later) in the hospital's high-level TBI program and had daily occupational (OT), physical (PT), and speech-language pathology (SLP) therapies. First my notes read, in the handwriting of my therapists Chelsea, Ashley, and Mary Ellen:

> Tuesday, Sept. 4, 2012
> 7:30–8:30 OT Chelsea
> - Played Connect Four
> - Worked on organization/visual spatial tasks
> 9:30–10:30 SLP Ashley
> - Worked on reading
> - Finding words
> - Putting stories in order
> 2:00–2:45 PT Mary Ellen
> - Worked on pathfinding on the rehab unit, finding your way to the dining room, gym + back to your room
> - Walked while kicking soccer ball forward + backward. You did great on your balance

I'm sure I bored Mary Ellen to tears with stories about playing Division I soccer in college and coaching in high school the year before my injury. Those memories fueled my recovery—I yearned to recapture that active lifestyle. Because of this journal, I know that my wife and son were scheduled to visit me the next day, September 5, though I don't remember it now. Some of what's noted from that time in the journal, I do remember—but not much.

I remember trying to do the math on my first day of therapy, we moved to simple arithmetic and I knew numbers but I had no idea what the symbol + signified. Chelsea explained that meant I should add together the numbers, and that it was okay to count out the progressive values. In this way, I moved from counting "seven to eight to nine" and all the way to fifteen for 7 + 8. I remember feeling a sense of wonder and achievement. This was fascinating. It was a challenge, no question, and I was up for it. I knew I worked at a high school—I *knew* that, I *remembered*—and I knew I should be there right now for the start of school. *Wait, oh shit, how did I miss the start of school?* I remember thinking. I was so attuned to deadlines—my life was structured around never missing deadlines, that had been ingrained in my professional life in publishing—that I was filled with a panic feeling about being in the hospital. However, that would soon change to immense gratitude after I better understood the nature of my injury.

Early in September, my writer friends Karl and Nancy were allowed to visit me, as Nancy is a pediatric nurse and is likely known in medical circles in northwestern Vermont; she also lives and works in the Burlington area. Visits to this rehabilitation-care facility were discouraged or not allowed, at least not the former soccer players I had coached in high school or coworkers or friends. My brother had come to see me in August, which I did not remember (it was during my period of amnesia)—except for the lingering feeling of a loving presence being with me. I had powerful dreams of water and fishing, as I've already mentioned. I'm bothered to this day by the hazy memory of a writing dream I had that I thought was very real at that time in September 2012—David Foster Wallace was a part of it, even though I'm not a big fan of his writing. When my boss came to visit me at the hospital (my wife told the doctors that would be okay), I mentioned something about the theme of that dream and some writing on which I was working, like I had some secret, privileged information. I'm sure it was nonsense, I think it was about entering a writing-award competition, maybe even the Pulitzer Prize? Could've been the Nobel. I remember it seemed very important. There was probably a lot of nonsense coming from me at that time. I have a record of emailing my boss at the school on September 12, one of my first sneaky emails from the hospital's common-area PC in the cafeteria: "Any email forwards I should see?" I wrote. I know I worked hard at that note, avoiding typos and being as deliberate and specific with my keyboard strokes as I could be. Maybe the automatic address function in Hotmail filled in his email address, because I could not have recalled it at that stage.

My memory of visitors is of taking a walk outside the hospital with Karl and Nancy, enjoying the Indian summer day in September, seeing the leaves blush with the dawn of autumn and the aroma of freshly cut grass. Karl told me recently we never left my hospital floor—we never went outside. I asked them to describe the visit, and Karl wrote to me:

"Nancy insisted we get you a present, so on our way to Fanny Allen Rehab where you had been consigned until you made sense again, we stopped at a book store and found two blank journal books and a colorful pen or two. 'He's a writer,' Nancy reminded me. 'He can write in these,' said Nancy. 'He probably has a lot to say.' You did. When you saw the notebooks you said, 'What are these?'"

I still have the Moleskine notebooks, Karl and Nancy. I've written in them since, sensibly! Karl continued in his note about not seeing me be me:

When we arrived in his room, we saw he was not alone. Sitting on a chair in the corner was his keeper or watcher, whom I recall looked like a fourteen-year-old and who kept his eyes on Joe all the time. Joe was dressed, sitting up on his bed. There were books around him, get-well cards on the wall, and he greeted us with "Hello, Nancy! Hello, Karl!" But I think that was right after we said, "Hi, Joe, I'm Nancy" and "Hi, Joe, I'm Karl." There were a couple of times in the course of conversation when he narrowed his eyes, furrowed his brow, and looked at us with a who-on-earth-are-these-people look. This is a very clear recollection of mine—Joe going from presenting a very relaxed aspect to one of rather grim alarm or concern—maybe confusion. I think this bothered me the most, for I was, naturally, looking for clues of understanding and continuity.

But the big surprise came as we left. Joe got out of bed, said he'd walk with us to the elevator. Watcher boy rose. We walked out of his room, down the corridor, pushed the down button, and Joe said, "I'm so glad you've come for me. I'm all set to go." Watcher boy closed in with, "Joe, you are staying, your guests are going."

Joe said, "No," and moved toward the elevator. Clearly he was confused and maybe a bit angry—as if we had tricked him, thwarted a foreordained plan to go home. Nancy explained to Joe he was not leaving, gave him a hug, and that seemed to mollify him a bit, but I shall never forget that look in his face as we stood in the elevator as the doors closed: Like that of a prisoner who was at the gate of release only to be told, "There's been a ghastly mistake. You have ten more years to serve." Confusion, sorrow, and even a bit of fear. Or maybe it was I, afraid for him.

I do remember Karl and Nancy coming to visit me and they were familiar to me but I'm not sure I remembered their names, and I also remember an awkward moment at the elevator, when I thought I would keep walking with them, leaving the hospital. I somehow knew a fast-food place was across the street from the hospital, I had noticed it on a walk outside with a therapist or I had seen it from a window. Leaving the hospital seemed very important and I was determined to do so, until I saw it was hopeless—"watcher boy" as Karl writes was a male nurse assigned to me—at which point I returned to my hospital bed and probably fell asleep, as I'm sure I was exhausted from the visit.

Soon after—it could've been the next morning's therapy session, it could have already happened the day before—a therapist placed a card in front of me showing seven x eight and immediately I knew the answer was fifty-six. I needed no explanation of what x signified, the product simply popped into my head. As simple as that surely sounds, it was the moment when I knew—*I knew deeply*—that I would be okay. I've always hated math, my entire life I've thought of it as superfluous, yet here the knowledge (or ingrained memory, from elementary school) brought an internal sense of reassurance that I would be okay. This sudden ability to recognize a simple math calculation impelled me on to the next challenges in recovery, such as deduction exercises, logic and reasoning, and word-finding puzzles.

I know this: I had a powerful drive to do well, I wanted to be a model student, to make the honor roll, to join the National Head Trauma Honor

Society, to master every challenge. I suppose I did okay, because I was released after a couple of weeks, on September 17. Without fanfare, of course. I've learned since that time that our insurance was still active—a couple of months after my release, it dawned on me that maybe I was discharged from the hospital because our insurance was maxed out, but that wasn't the case. I was ready. I simply went home with my wife. After a national-chain restaurant lunch—Friendly's, I think—and a grocery-shopping stop, I was so happy to be home. The familiar smells, the moody way the autumnal light played through the windows, my hunting dog— even the black cat! I was back. I went to our bed and curled up in the fresh-scent sheets to take a nap.

The ensuing weeks went by uneventfully. My wife explained that I was on disability from work and I could not contact the office. My right arm was still in a cast. I was banged up and visibly needed to heal. I would be having surgery at Dartmouth-Hitchcock Medical Center in November, my wife told me, to repair the wrist. That was the physical—but the unseen was the larger challenge.

I was free to relax, sleep, and read. I heard a radio promotion for Lumosity.com so went to that URL, joined, and started an online program of brain training with a focus on memory, attention, and problem solving. I had my MacBook Pro from work and my four-year-old son played with me. We teamed up on *Pinball Recall, Lost in Migration, Familiar Faces*, and *Eagle Eye*—my son was quick! I treasured spending the time with him, as we both worked at our cognitive footholds, him for the first time in life and me in my effort to reestablish my brain skills.

My good friend Peter Miller (go to www.silverprintpress.com to see his work), a talented photographer and writer based near Stowe, Vermont, with whom I worked at *Vermont Magazine* years before this turn in my life, was organizing his life's work of photography and narrative profiles into the large-format hardcover book *A Lifetime of Vermont People* and I now had the time to help. I had been reviewing a batch of Peter's digital photos on the day of my accident, looking for autumn shots for a calendar I was planning to produce to promote the high school in 2013, as I had done for the school in 2011 for the year 2012. Peter had worked at

Life magazine as a reporter, after assisting the famed photographer Yousuf Karsh in Europe. Karsh's photographs of Ernest Hemingway, Humphrey Bogart, Andy Warhol, JFK, and more of that era's celebrities are widely known. Peter developed his own signature black-and-white photographic style, as seen in such excellent books as *Vermont People* and *Vermont Farm Women*. I offered to donate my editorial time and Peter accepted and asked his art director to email me galley PDFs of pages from his book layout, which I would edit and proofread and send back to "Cookie," as Peter affectionately called his art director. I was overjoyed to be working on the book; I felt it was the absolute perfect cognitive therapy for me.

As I told Peter in 2013, today I feel this focus and engagement was a major contributor to regaining my abilities as quickly as I did; the intensive study of his photos and more the proof reading of his writing presented on the page heightening my cognitive acuity, reestablishing pathways I had developed through decades of writing and editing—reconnecting neurons in Wernicke's and Broca's areas, firing together again in harmony, joyously. (This felt like a karmic connection between Peter and me.) He had sent me a letter when he learned of my fall, which I saw when I got home from the hospital. He wrote a free-verse poem about the "Helldamn cat!" and included the narrative of "Walking in Beauty: Closing Prayer from the Navajo Way Blessing Ceremony."

Peter, a lifelong fly fisherman and wingshooter, wrote of the poem: "It is very apt for people like you and me. We have found this beauty in love for women and children. We have seen it while on the beach at dawn and dusk, deciphering the waves and currents, in an old apple orchard on a wet fall day, the grouse there, somewhere, your dog all stiff-legged, creeping forward. Or that moment when the dog is in the alders, locked on point, a woodcock about to spiral up but where? There! The full moon in November, rising as a silver disk behind a maple skinned of leaves, the thin branches like veins across the moon's surface. The thin bubble of a rise at the edge of the stream, the water blue as the sky, the current slow, and a breeze so light on which floats the perfume of wild flowers . . . a moose and a calf walking down-stream below you, above the rapids."

I'm a spiritual brother of Peter's, from another generation perhaps, but we have similar outlooks on life—including the propensity to begin to feel put upon or impatient with the, quote-unquote, normal masses. Our work is what matters, sometimes all that matters. His words to me were reassuring and, the more I read them, enlivening. The work on his book, offered to me as a focus and occupation during those months of recovery, was a salvation. Working on his book saved me. It saved my identity of who I am and what I believe my value in life to be. I embraced and edited each chapter I received in galleys from the art director. It was fun. All the gloom that had distressed my vision—all the imagined crud accumulated in my brain's gyri or sulci—was gone. I now loved life—I love life *now*. In his letter, Peter quoted the Navajo poem:

> Today I walk out, today everything negative will leave me
> I will be as I was before, I will have a cool breeze over my body.
> I will have a light body, I will be happy forever, nothing will
> > Hinder me.
> I walk in beauty before me. I walk with beauty behind me.
> I walk with beauty below me. I walk with beauty above me.
> I walk with beauty around me. My words will be beautiful.
> > In beauty all day long may I walk.
> Through the returning seasons, may I walk.
> On the trail marked with pollen, may I walk.
> > With dew about my feet, may I walk.
> > With beauty before me may I walk.
> > With beauty behind me may I walk.
> > With beauty below me may I walk.
> > With beauty above me may I walk.
> > With beauty all around me may I walk.
> In old age wandering on a trail of beauty. Lively, may I walk.
> In old age wandering on a trail of beauty, living again, may I walk.
> > My words will be beautiful . . .

Peter's inspiring letter was waiting for me in a stack of wonder-ful, incredible cards from people dear and important in my life, some of whom I had not thought about in far too long. I was stunned. As I was still only vaguely aware of the severity of my accident, I was astounded people would write to me. The sheer emotional purity of writing, the unadulterated expression—there it was, stacked up. Not emails or voice messages, but cards and letters. I realized again then how lucky I was in life, undeserving but lucky to have people who cared this much in my life.

That day, I needed to sleep, which I did often during those first months of recovery. I had been given the gift of time by an insurance provider making the disability benefit real. I could recover in my own time.

I had a visitor at home then, a good friend from the high school, an English teacher who just had her first novel published, Jennifer Land. She stopped by on her way to a book reading at the school, I think it was, and we sat on my deck looking south at the sun's reflection glinting off the observation tower or the Tram House on Cannon Mountain. Her book, which I highly recommend, is *The Spare Room*, set during the time of the Underground Railroad in pre-Civil War Vermont. The publishers, Neil Raphel and Janis Raye, are also friends. (St. Johnsbury is a small town.) Jenny's book offers insight into why Vermont is and always has been a special state and state of mind. I couldn't express much to Jenny at that time, I only could emote appreciation for her being with me. My publishing friend Phil Monahan also came by and I was a little stronger then, cognitively. We worked together editing fly-fishing magazines and he was an astute editorial voice reading my attempts at fiction years before. We've also enjoyed fishing together, particularly off the coast of Massachusetts and in the Rocky Mountains, and he tolerated me struggling to train my first bird dog as we hunted together. Phil is now a promotional writer for The Orvis Company in Vermont. As I wrote in Chapter 4, my sister Jennifer visited from California. In November, I had surgery on my right arm. My parents came from Florida for Thanksgiving.

I needed time and I needed support, throughout these months. The dormitory staff at the high school brought a team of boarding students to stack my firewood. I'm happy to say I do that work myself now. The twelve full cords of firewood in my yard are the evidence. I was cleared to drive again by an occupational therapist at Dartmouth-Hitchcock Medical Center (my license was never revoked but could have been, and in any case neither my wife nor the doctors would have permitted me to drive if I exhibited symptoms of severe cognitive impairment); I wasn't required by the state to have a driving assessment, as some patients are. I began to talk with a clinical therapist about my emotions and I met with another for cognitive outpatient therapy once a week at the nearby regional hospital. I had started this outpatient therapy a week after I got home, working with a speech therapist once a week on cognitive and vocational efforts at the hospital in New Hampshire.

"You definitely had trouble with word retrieval, organization, your verbal output was very slow; you were searching for words, you didn't quite know how to put words together, sometimes, and how to say them. But your expressive capabilities were quite good," said Jennifer Scianna, the therapist with whom I worked. When I interviewed Jen while writing this book, I reminded her I remembered neither the accident nor the subsequent three weeks of hospitalization, and she said that's common—"That's one thing about head injury, everybody says the same thing, that they just don't remember that period in the hospital. It's not usually until people get home in their familiar environments again that they really start to make better memories, it's like 'Okay, I'm more in my element now, it's very familiar to me.' It's difficult in a hospital setting because there's nothing familiar around you so it doesn't call up memory and you're relying on raw memory. Whereas, when you get home you have more context," she told me. I found this true to my experience.

I asked her how she and other therapists decide on a course of recovery action for patients with brain injury. "A lot of it's based on what patients' final goals are, what they want to get back to, what they consider their baseline. A lot of the therapies we pick and choose depend on what your goals are. The family's big in those early stages, too. Like finding out if this is reliable information the patient is giving me, because you can't always know if the patient's memory is working correctly," Jen said. Jen talked with my wife, from time to time, during that early period. She further told me,

> By the time you got here, your insight was fairly good. You were scared. You were scared you would not be able to get back to work. You saw your limitations much better than most people. You saw, "Oh, jeez, I'm not going to be able to handle all that stuff. I'm not going to be able to focus, I'm not going to be able to read and write like I did." You were nervous about it. One of the places we almost always begin with head injury is attention and concentration, so we did start with that with you, as well. You would tend to be easily distracted by things in the environment. So it was getting basic exercises, where you had to attend, and you might get off track but I would watch and ask myself *Can he draw himself back?* That's a big step for everything, because if you can't attend and you can't concentrate, you're not going to get very far.

I mentioned to Jen how I learned to attend, over time, through meditation—I learned the value of being in the moment and being present in the now. She agreed that meditation is valuable:

> It's a really hard thing, to not have thoughts dart at you—I even have a hard time at that, to not think about my grocery list.
>   So we started on attention and concentration and then we moved on to organization and sequencing. A job like yours [at the time] required a lot of organization and sequencing. Also memory strategies, how and what's going to work best for you to remember appointments and get your independence. How can you track your own schedule without having

someone else do it all the time? We worked on calendars and lists—and especially to-do lists. Anything that you needed to remember, we wrote down. We did some journal writing, for basic memory and organizational thoughts. That's important, organizational tasks like "What am I going to do today?" and writing that down.

We next moved to reading comprehension and organization—taking information and categorizing it in the proper order. Jen said my verbal reasoning was pretty good—Broca's and Wernicke's areas were quickly responding—so our next endeavor was to play games, first having me explain the rules to Jen so I would begin to understand myself. I took the board game Rummikub seriously, I remember that, and worked to master laying down the melds so all of the tiles on my player's board were placed on the table in sequence. These patterns of organization and sequencing were outstanding exercises. As Jen recalled:

> A lot of those games, and you probably didn't realize it at the time, required attention and concentration. We would add background noises, as time went on, so you had to pay attention to what you were doing, weed out the background noise, and then had tasks that required divided attention. You might have been doing one thing, and you had to sequence something over here, and then you had to visually scan. We did a lot of those types of activities.

Jen is referring to manufactured distractions, as I call them. This was part of working memory—in which you're manipulating memory in your head and holding on to thoughts and calculations to get to a conclusion of another kind, Jen said. It can be a skill as simple as adding numbers in your head.

Jen recalled that during one therapy session, near my return to work, I told her I thought I was getting worse. She said that my insight and awareness were in fact getting better. "You were nervous about the few limitations you still may have had," she said.

"Organization, sequencing—and flexibility. The left side (of the brain) and executive function skills, these were the ones you were really working on," Jen said. "You were there (in your abilities), you just needed to get back and do it," Jen said. "You just needed to get back to work." That was far and away my goal—the ultimate return to normalcy, to me, equated returning to work.

I had seen a doctor at the rehab hospital around this time, which resulted in a casual challenge to write this book, if I was able. The doctor also judged that I wasn't yet ready to return to work and would need an examination by a neuropsychologist and neuropsychological testing. (Detailed in Chapter 3, my interaction with Dr. Matthew Kraybill.)

I asked Hannah Deene Wood for thoughts on recovery from her TBI. "Advice to loved ones? It's gotta be time. Slow down, just give them time." Easier said than done, she also admitted. "I was like, 'I want it now, I want to be better now!'"

I told her, after two years (as I write this), I still want it now. She said she does, too, after almost thirteen years from the time of her injury when we spoke. "Because we live in this McDonald's society, we all want everything to happen so fast," she said. "I think with my brain injury, it's gone in peaks and valleys. I've gone through weird slumps. I've had deep depression and that's part of a brain injury," Hannah said. "Not that my path has been so nasty, because it hasn't been," she continued. She owns a skate park in Vermont and is surrounded by the brightness of youth. She said:

> I escape through Zumba—it saved my life. I needed some women in my life, because skateboarding is all about little boys and their dads bringing the little boys to skateboard. Now that's changing, girls are coming and that's great. But I needed something to get me feeling alive. I went into a Zumba class, and the music started, and you have to move your body to the beat. That is so good for the brain. I became addicted to it. Everybody

loves music and music is so healing and brings out a picture of that inner joy.

Hanna has a strong personality and has dedicated herself to helping other TBI patients. "I get letters and I got one from a mom in California and she talked about how mad and angry her son is and I said, 'Embrace that! He's alive! He's telling you, 'I've *got* this.' What's the alternative? Embrace it, it's okay, give him time," said Hannah.

When I woke up after my injury, I was filled with inner joy. That was burning to emerge before I climbed the ladder; I was searching for a foothold in life, as I knew I was living an unfulfilling existence but I couldn't stop or change my behavior. One winter's day about six months before my fall, on my lunch hour from the high school, I took a drive and wound up on Interstate 91 approaching Barnet, Vermont. I took the Barnet exit and stopped at Karmê Chöling Shambhala Center, for more than forty years one of the main Shambhala meditation centers in the world. The earth's energy pulled me there. I took a walk on the campus, down to the river that runs through the land, and felt I could be helped and healed there. Months before, I was introduced to the executive director, Jane Arthur, and was intrigued by the work being done at the center. When Melissa Jenkins, the teacher and coworker at my workplace, was murdered in March 2012, I was caught in a dizzying emotional spiral. Now my core self was seeking to move into the operator's seat of my consciousness.

I was cleared to return to work in mid-January 2013. I guess I had made the honor roll in recovery, after all.

I continued cognitive therapy and emotional-conversational therapy, feeling more and more secure with my sense of self. The school was past midterm, into the exciting months of denouement for the 200-plus seniors graduating that June. I worked out in the school's weight room on my strength and continued working on my overall health. My perception is that I got through the semester, with help and support from my colleagues, including a former private-school headmaster, John Suitor, who shouldered much of the marketing administrative management during those months. This support carried me along, into a summer program for incoming freshmen, in which I was asked to teach the basics of marketing and customer relations to eager "rising freshmen," as the cohort of incoming ninth-grade students is called.

I discovered another form of therapy around this time—the value of basic, goal-oriented, repetitive hard work like splitting and stacking wood or cutting the lawn. The day before high school graduation that year, before the school's baccalaureate ceremony for seniors, I got a panicked phone call from my wife that trees had fallen on our house. Sure enough, a wind shear had raged along our ridge property and uprooted a couple of ash and rock-maple trees, felling them against our house. The branches did minor damage to the roof, but more providentially we had our firewood for the next winter. I bought a log splitter and spent the next few months splitting and stacking wood, about eight full cords. In 2014, I started the firewood preparation in May and split and stacked about twelve full cords, allowing them to season throughout the summer. This is not challenging work, and that's the value—you work toward a goal of, say, splitting a cord a week and then you have the 128-cubic-feet pile to stack over another few days. The repetition allows the mind to wander, and for me that's freeing. You can be present when you need to be—when you're operating the hydraulic splitting wedge, for example—and let your mind go at other times. I find this to be true of running a push mower to cut the lawn in spring and summer, shoveling snow in the winter, and raking leaves in fall. Which makes me appreciate the seasonal beauties of living in Vermont, all the more. I've already mentioned deliberate pursuits like fly fishing and bird hunting providing the same mental escapes and foci outside myself—these are all transformational. I know it's a matter of looking at the activities a certain way, now with appreciation and curiosity.

A year after my injury, at the start of the fall 2013 semester, during another faculty "in service" meeting preparing for the return of students from the summer break, a social studies teacher talked to the staff and faculty about mindfulness meditation and invited those interested to take part in before-school group meditation sessions. I mention this because it was a vital experience for my recovery and I now believe that meditation is a pathway to healing for everyone—and particularly for brain-injury survivors. We can aid in the retraining of our brains, through meditation. We can quiet the internal clatter and tumult in our minds—or the nattering internal monologue criticizing, beseeching, scolding, cajoling. I'm living proof.

Mindfulness acquainted me with the simple idea of being curious about my own thoughts, appreciating them, and allowing them to dwell within my head without conflict—simply to be curious about the thoughts emanating from my own mind.

By focusing on your own breath in and out, you can calm and quiet your thoughts and therefore regulate your mental existence. This is the new consciousness I found—to appreciate and partner with my thoughts, not to antagonize myself or to constantly analyze or be in perpetual conflict with my thoughts and therefore myself. Peace and contentment are fundamental ideas of mindfulness meditation. When I was part of a seminar at Karmê Chöling later in my recovery, one participant described this calming as "the sediment settling in roily water." The knowledge was that my own thoughts were transitory, like bluefish in a bait-feeding frenzy, all sound and fury signifying nothing.

I found the morning mindfulness sessions at the school restful and emancipating—an oasis in a frantic atmosphere, as a high school is a churning, distractive place and marketing an international boarding school (it was more like a small college than a high school) happened at a relentless and unruly pace. My therapy sessions also gave me the opening to talk about angst and feelings of being different from the pre-injury me. Having time and open space to talk helped me, and developed the accompanying appreciation that I wasn't alone in this world and didn't have to face (and fight) this life alone.

The love that I received during my hospitalization created an emotional flood tide inside me. As my brain reestablished neural pathways, my emotions reordered to be more receptive to feelings and able to transmit them. My limbic system was functioning differently (or some of the individual parts, like the hippocampus and amygdala, perhaps, were)—maybe now firing and wiring together in harmony. I had grown as an adult with a head injury beyond the guardedness I had learned as a child in a reticent family in which we collectively harbored and contained our emotions.

I feel I've always been an empathetic individual, but what I was feeling, emoting, and receiving in my recovery was different from pure empathy—it was more complete, more self-possessing, deeper, and brought an ease over me. It was the real experience of the four essentials, the Divine Abidings—Compassion, Joy, Love, Equanimity—shown on the amulet I wear around my neck, nestled into my being. The brightest of the four is equanimity, a high *jhana* path, I've learned, in Buddhist traditions—pure and distilled clarity. Now I was in touch with that. My recovery was going much deeper than I ever imagined, blossoming outward, or perhaps reaching higher to an elevated awareness—truly to a new consciousness.

Meditation helped me advance through my recovery by allowing me to maintain control of my consciousness. Jane Arthur of Karmê Chöling had simple thoughts about this: "This is an approach that's not living in your reruns." She said we all have groups of thoughts that are habituated—we are caught in the past, or caught up in regret or fantasy; our thoughts just as readily go to the future—and steal our minds from the present moment.

"We have to rehabituate ourselves to a different way of being with our own minds. Our natural minds contain a huge amount of wisdom and compassion and space. We've been trained by our culture to disregard this. We have little curiosity. But it's a great place to start, to be curious—you could open your mind just a little bit to the possibility of being curious," she told the class at Karmê Chöling during a weekend retreat on wakefulness and appreciation called "Relax, Renew, Awaken."

"How do we get back to the mind that has peacefulness, is a source of wisdom and kindness and compassion, and deep clarity? There is not a human being who does not have this. How do we get back to it? How do we have a mind—what I call our human equipment—open to possibility? It's not that far away and it's peeking up all the time. We're not just working with calming ourselves, but working toward a fuller, more feeling life," Jane said to the class by way of introducing meditation. "If we weren't supposed to feel, why did we get this equipment, this ability to feel?"

We are, after all, *homo sapiens sapiens*—they who know, and know that they know. We have the ability of language and are able to use complex tools, including our brain. Our own brain is mutable and plastic and we can change its function, and therefore our behavior, by training our neurons to wire and fire together, opening new neural pathways. This is not a high-minded concept—neuroscientists have proved it to be real.

"Preparing the mind begins with stopping for a moment to see what our mind feels like," wrote Sakyong Mipham in *Turning the Mind Into An Ally*. Simply noticing and appreciating our thoughts allows us to slow down. "Speed kills," Jane Arthur further said. "It makes our world aggressive and unkind, we're moving so fast, it's almost like the drug of this particular time is speed. We haven't been taught to meditate. Or we haven't grown up in a culture that frankly valued it," she said to the weekend class that I attended.

Later, when I spoke with her one-on-one in a local bookstore in St. Johnsbury, Vermont, she said, "I think meditation is the most potent way one could spend a short period of time. If you don't have a lot of time, it's going to pay off. That's the pith of it. Just try it. It's a tradition that goes back a very long time, it's part of all mystical, deep, profound traditions. It's a human activity, not a religious activity. It's as old as time."

This counters the preconception (a mistaken one, of course) that meditation is Buddhist by definition or imbued with religious intent. It is a *secular* method of channeling the power of our minds, of organizing at least some number of the eighty-five billion or more neurons firing in our individual brains—it can create a sort of meta–executive function process in the brain, in which organization, planning, strategizing, paying attention, and managing time and space all are directed toward the good. We can channel and harness the power of our minds for positive outcomes—that is, *basic goodness*, to invoke the term used in the Shambhala Buddhist tradition. Achieving peaceful abiding through gentle attention to our thoughts is what this type of meditation intends.

Jane Arthur also told me, you really can't learn this through a book— and as a beginner to meditation, I have to agree, though everyone does have to start with a guide and in the absence of personal human instruction a book serves as a beginning. It's an individual, humanistic process, just like recovery from brain injury. Everyone approaches the process differently, from different directions and with different individualized intent, we bring our own measure of self and we can adjust who we are, if we want to. That said, Sakyong Mipham Rinpoche offers help in *Turning the Mind Into An Ally* through "Instructions for Contemplative Meditation":

1. Calm the mind by resting on the breathing.
2. When you feel ready, bring up a certain thought or intention in the form of words.
3. Use these words as the object of meditation, continually returning to them as distractions arise.

Sakyong Mipham recommends creating a "heartfelt experience" by conjuring meaning in the word or words and letting that provide inspiration. You'll use that feeling of inspiration to let the words slip away and dwell in that feeling. This is restful, but don't be tempted to let the feeling deepen and carry you off to sleep. You should be relaxed, and by focusing on your breath you maintain that relaxation and steady rhythm. The breath is your somatic connection.

He also instructs: "Conclude your session and arise from your meditation with the meaning in your heart. 'Meaning' is direct experience, free of words."

Know that "sakyong" means earth protector in Tibetan and is the designation given to the leader of the Shambhala lineage, as Mipham is, as was his father Chögyam Trungpa Rinpoche; his father is credited with founding Shambhala and he also founded Karmê Chöling in Barnet, Vermont, and the contemplative university Naropa Institute, now Naropa University based in Boulder, Colorado. His teachings are recorded in *The Collected Works of Chögyam Trungpa* from Shambhala Publications. In the book *The Shambhala Principle*, Sakyong Mipham the son says his father's teachings brought forth two simple ideas common to teachings of the Buddha, Plato, Aristotle, Jesus, Lao Tzu, Confucius, and also Judaism and Islam: "Humanity is good, and good is the nature of society."

Jane Arthur describes the process of opening up to meditation as courting oneself. "When you take ten minutes a day to meditate, it's like checking in with a lover. Courtship is the ongoing nature of getting to know someone. And we never court ourselves. I love the old-fashioned meaning of that word."

"Let me not to the marriage of true minds admit impediments," Shakespeare wrote in Sonnet 116, love is an ever-fixed mark. To find love inside of us means we have to let it out, allow it to emanate. This is the way to basic goodness and peaceful abiding. When we work to regain cognition, what a gift in life to work on regaining a cognition that has found itself in basic goodness.

The human brain is abundant with promise. It is magical. It is the ultimate equipment. That we can shape our awareness and direct our consciousness is the fullness of life. It can start with ten minutes a day. The exploration can begin inside all of us. The fullness of intentional behavior is the result.

We are human—all we can do is try.

Our brains are our human equipment, about which we continue to learn more and more each passing year. The attention gained from the 2014 Nobel Prize in Physiology or Medicine going to noted neuroscientists John O'Keefe, May Britt-Moser, and Edvard I. Moser is one example of the fascination with brain function translated into scientific recognition of the highest order. To be sure, that we have gained greater scientific understanding of how we navigate complex environments is exciting knowledge—through the hippocampus, O'Keefe et al. discovered—and scientists now have a better grasp of brain maps and "place cells," but we're also learning more about effects and outcomes of brain injury, either from immediate trauma like falling off a ladder, or from repeated collisions in athletics, or traumatic injury, or experiencing traumatic events in warfare.

Our bodies have evolved a miraculous design and an astounding skeletal structure that foremost protects the brain. Let's honor, nurture, and cherish what the writer Kurt Vonnegut called "the crowning glory of evolution"—the human brain.

II

CURRENT BRAIN EXPLORATION AND POTENTIAL PATHWAYS TO RECOVERY

When it comes to study of the human brain—probing scientific examination leading to empirical discovery and physiological, bio-medical, and neuroscientific knowledge—today's neurologists and neuroscientists are Christopher Columbus in lab coats. Their work launches them into the great unknown, a fantastic voyage into our organic super computer; their achievements are in the spirit of Copernicus, Magellan, Einstein, or Lewis and Clark, or perhaps even Captain James T. Kirk, striving to boldly go where no one has yet been, in knowledge and understanding.

The same type of exploration undertaken by these personages in history is under way as directed by physicians and scientists, focused back on us as a species and "the mystery of the three pounds of matter that sits between our ears," as President Barack Obama said in April 2013 when he announced the project launched under his tenure called the BRAIN Initiative. The acronym BRAIN stands for Brain Research through Advancing Innovative Neurotechnologies, and Obama's hope was that we would benefit as a culture from advancing our collective understanding of brain function. Hundreds of millions of dollars in federal, foundation, and corporate funding have been promised to benefit the program. Gaining better understanding of the brain should lead to greater knowledge of Parkinson's, Alzheimer's, Traumatic Brain Injury, epilepsy, PTSD, schizophrenia, depression, and other brain disorders and neurologic diseases. And better understanding of neurologic maladies perhaps will lead to treatments.

Though announced in 2013, the program so far has been lightly reported in the media, and therefore remains a reference known mainly in the corridors of science centers and laboratories, kind of inside baseball for neurologists and those seeking neurology-related grant funding. However, the knowledge and inevitable discoveries of the ten-year program—the duration presently is set for 2016 to 2025—could potentially yield tremendous advances in humanistic understanding.

Certainly, the increased knowledge of the brain and its pathways leading to function may create more cultural sensitivity and compassion for those with neurologic difficulties, impairments, and injuries. Obama has stated that his administration also expects economic boosts from the study of the brain, as is the shared goal of all Grand Challenge programs of his administration. The message is that innovation leads to a stronger economy.

A report from the BRAIN Initiative Working Group to the National Institutes of Health Director stated, "Through deepened knowledge of how our brains actually work, we will understand ourselves differently, treat disease more incisively, educate our children more effectively, practice law and governance with greater insight, and develop more understanding of others whose brains have been molded in different circumstances." The timeline from 2016 to 2025, the report reads, will begin "with a primary focus on technology development in the first five years, shifting in the second five years to a primary focus on integrating technologies to make fundamental new discoveries about the brain."

Understanding brain circuits is cited as an initial area of examination, along with identifying the various cells at work in the brain and their functions, and how synaptic connections occur between circuits and systems in the brain. The investigations of the brain will be paired with technologies available to scientists now—MRIs, fMRIs, electroencephalography (EEG), magnetoencephalography (MEG), positron emission tomography (PET scans), and the like—and emerging and future neurotechnologies, with the intent to produce a working map of the functioning brain. This may lead to the discovery of new forms of neural coding, the report also states. The focus on neural circuitry may shed light on how neurotransmitters (biological chemicals) and synapses (electrical impulses) work in concert throughout the 80 to 100 billion neurons and glial cells in our brain to create thoughts, emotions, aspirations, desires, perceptions, and memories, leading to behaviors.

"The BRAIN Initiative is primarily focused on developing new tools. The National Institutes of Health (NIH) dedicates five and-a-half billion dollars to neuroscience research every year on depression, schizophrenia, Alzheimer's, Parkinson's, epilepsy, TBI—hundreds of different disorders of the nervous system. We have lots of people working hard on how these disorders can be attenuated or ameliorated. But we can't make progress if we don't have the right tools. The right types of tools can either interrogate or modulate the circuits in the brain," said Dr. Walter Koroshetz, acting director, National Institute of Neurological Disorders and Stroke (NINDS) with a leadership role in the NIH's BRAIN Initiative. I interviewed Dr. Koroshetz in December 2014.

"There's a lot of enthusiasm but also a lot of frustration about getting the right tools. There's a war on these diseases and you want to go into it with the most powerful weapons. Right now, we're still in the bow-and-arrow stage," Dr. Koroshetz continued. "The brain is a super computer, it's all based on circuits. Circuits for breathing, moving, sensing. We know the circuits exist, but we don't have good ways of measuring the activity of the circuits. The tools we have now are things like EEG and brainwave tests—kind of like a line cartoon compared to a Monet. It's a very crude sampling of what's actually going on in the brain circuits. What we'd like to do is figure out ways to see how the cells are actually firing. We've been doing that, but only seeing one cell and not the entire circuit, which might have one hundred million cells. So we'd like to figure out ways in which we can record tens of thousands of cells firing simultaneously, and actually see the cells lighting up, so we can see the critical pattern because we think it's the pattern that's the key to the function of the circuit. We don't really have a good way of doing that now."

The Working Group report states, simply: "Our charge is to understand the circuits and patterns of neural activity that give rise to mental experience and behavior." According to Dr. Koroshetz, this study has begun in genetically modified primitive organisms, such as zebra fish and mice. "We've placed genes in a mouse so you shine a light into the brain and the cells light up. This is called optogenetics, a way to interrogate the nervous system of the organism, interrogating the circuits and asking, How does that lead to behavior? In zebra fish, scientists can link the circuitry to the behavior, like feeding, and can see the active areas of the brain light up. That will show us the causal nature of how it all happens," the doctor said. Next might come similar studies in primates such as marmosets, he added.

"We really want to learn about the human brain, so we're working our way up from non-human primates and then we'll look at humans. We're working from the bottom up and the top in, with techniques that are non-invasive but recording circuitry in the brain," Dr. Koroshetz said—like blood flow changing in the brain as shown on an fMRI image once cells begin firing. "When part of the brain activates, yes, neurotransmitters are released, but the brain cells fire and they need more energy—they're like little electrical circuits—so they need more blood flow. Channels open, ions flow in, there's a need for more blood flow to meet the metabolic need," he said. "The trouble is, fMRI is slow. Changes happen so fast, and this is about five hundred times too slow," he continued. "Spatially, the resolution is not that great. We need techniques that measure something that's changing faster. The question is, what's next?"

Learning more about brain circuits will lead to more knowledge of the parts of the brain as a whole. "We're asking, What are the components? We hope to have a census of all the different types of cells, leading to a parts list of the brain," Dr. Koroshetz said. The BRAIN Initiative Working Paper states, "we must define the cellular components of circuits, including their molecular properties and anatomical connections. This knowledge will tell us what the brain is made of at molecular, cellular, and structural levels; it will also provide a foundation for understanding how these properties change across the normal lifespan and in brain disorders."

The Working Group Report further states, "it is no exaggeration to say that nothing in neuroscience makes sense except in the light of behavior. Thus a primary theme of the BRAIN Initiative should be to illuminate how the tens of billions of neurons in the central nervous system interact to produce behavior." A section of the Report continues: "Theory, modeling, and statistics will be essential to understanding the brain" and that the BRAIN Initiative team "must turn to theory, simulation, and sophisticated quantitative analysis in our search to understand the underlying mechanisms that bridge spatial and temporal scales, linking components and their interactions to the dynamic behavior of the intact system." Dr. Koroshetz acknowledges that this will take a lot of data and NIH scientists are looking to forge partnerships with information-management companies such as Google, Amazon, Intel, and others. The Working Group Report states,

With these increasingly powerful techniques come new data sets of massive size and complexity. Reconstructing neural circuits and their dynamic activity in fine detail will require image analysis at a formidable scale as well as simultaneous activity measurements from thousands of neurons. The age of "big data" for the brain is upon us. Thus, neuroscientists are seeking increasingly close collaborations with experts in computation, statistics, and theory in order to mine and understand the secrets embedded in their data. These startling new technologies, many of which did not exist ten years ago, force us to reconceive what it means to be an experimental neuroscientist today. The challenge that now faces neuroscience is to map the circuits of the brain, measure the fluctuating patterns of electrical and chemical activity flowing within those circuits, and understand how their interplay creates our unique cognitive and behavioral capabilities.

Dr. Koroshetz mentions how this increased understanding should lead to better pathways of recovery:

Scientists know how respiration and breathing works. But what's the equivalent when it comes to thinking or speaking? All we have is the output and the brain is a black box. You want to get inside the box and manipulate the important circuits. A lot of things have an effect on brain circuits. The brain is connected to the body, and there's a blood-brain barrier. The brain is controlling what gets across to it from the blood. There are controllers, like a firewall.

We do rehabilitation like cognitive behavior therapy, meditation, and we know we're changing the circuits but we don't know how we're doing it. We're kind of like shooting from the hip and walking in the dark. But we want to measure the change in the circuits so we can really focus the therapy. Recovery is ... you have a circuit that's been damaged and you're trying to get the circuit re-wired and back to functioning. We want to examine circuit function and use therapy to drive toward the good circuit function. That could be very powerful. We want a good circuit pattern in the end. We're always looking at the output, like kids learning math, but we never see the circuit. So that has to change. If you can't measure it, you can't fix it. It's really the final frontier of science, to understand the brain.

The body-brain connection is compelling to consider—particularly in recovery therapies, in which much of the work of cognitive recovery can be rote repetition and relearning, such as my own advancement from not recognizing the purpose of a plus sign to quickly knowing multiplication. Clearly, the circuits that were interrupted in my fall and resulting head injury began to reconnect and rewire and my memory returned, though slowly, over time. As I've written in this book, there was no medical panacea, I had to become familiar again with ideas and processes as the brain rewired. I could not take a pill—there was no chemical fix or faster recovery through drugs. Thanks to neuroplasticity, my brain began to heal itself and pathways reconnected as I reintroduced the puzzle pieces that would fit together to restore my cognitive function. Because my main injury occurred primarily to my left frontal lobe, my sequential and analytical skills took time to reestablish, and thankfully my linguistic skills came flooding back in the early months following my August 2012 fall.

My emotional brain—the thalamus, amygdala, hippocampus— seemed to be functioning intact and I certainly put more stock in them now than I did before my injury. I feel more emotionally balanced, in other words, since my injury, whereas prior to my fall I was much more rationally focused, perhaps due to a hyperactive prefrontal cortex.

I've been fascinated reading the work of Bessel van der Kolk, particularly his book *The Body Keeps the Score: Brain, Mind, and Body in the Healing of Trauma* and his discussion of bidirectional communication between body and mind. We know that evolution has allowed the body to regulate what substances enter the brain through blood flow and circulation. Alcohol, for example, readily passes into the brain system while some amino acids may not. But the brain is part of the nervous system so is affected by many chemicals carried in the blood and produced in the body, like serotonin, which is produced largely in the GI tract. The vagus nerve connects the heart, lungs, stomach, intestines, and the brain, so runs through the core of the human body. If the brain is our central processing unit (CPU), the vagus nerve would be our USB or Firewire, while the spinal cord is the multimedia interface cable. Dr. van der Kolk writes, "You can be fully in charge of your life only if you can acknowledge the reality of your body, in all its visceral dimensions . . . Being able to perceive visceral sensations is the very foundation of emotional awareness," which points out the need to connect viscerally with oneself in brain recovery, be it from PTSD or a traumatic experience such as molestation or rape or violent assault (including car accidents), or traumatic injury. Indeed, much of Dr. van der Kolk's clinical experience has been with recovery from many kinds of trauma. He writes about the value of yoga, the benefits of focusing on breathing during meditation (a way to regulate heart rate and generally slow down), mindfulness meditation, dialectical behavior therapy (DBT), EMDR (eye movement desensitization and reprocessing), internal family systems (IFS), and Pesso Boyden System Psychomotor therapy. "One of the clearest lessons from contemporary neuroscience is that our sense of ourselves is anchored in a vital connection with our bodies," Dr. van der Kolk writes in *The Body Keeps the Score*. "We do not truly know ourselves unless we can feel and interpret our physical sensations; we need to register and act on these sensations to navigate safely through life."

He also writes of alexithymia, or not being able to identify what is going on inside oneself, essentially becoming an empty vessel. This can make you detached and void of emotion—a real clinical concern for PTSD patients; but also of concern for brain-injury patients striving to regain a sense of normalcy and confidence in the ability to contribute to a job or to be a good parent, spouse, family member, or a functional member of society. This is a serious consideration in brain recovery—keeping the body in tune and aligned with the brain. Or keeping the two *allied and in balance*.

The dual practices of yoga and meditation unite the mind and the body. Both bring acceptance, appreciation leading to compassion, curiosity about what's happening with and within us, and ultimately somatic and cognitive unity. I strongly recommend both and personally have found meditation to be a tremendous boost in my new consciousness.

For example, the LoveYourBrain Foundation, cofounded by former professional snowboarder Kevin Pearce (who I've mentioned in this book, suffered a severe TBI while training for the Winter Olympics) has launched a yoga program for people with TBI. Their website reads, "Our goal is to support people with brain injury to strengthen and reconnect their mind and body through meditation and yoga." They recommend gentle and restorative yoga and meditation practices, as TBI recovery takes time and nurturing of oneself. Otherwise, depression is a risk. The group says that about a quarter of the people who suffer TBI report thinking about or attempting suicide. Yoga and meditation can curb this compulsion and ideation and allow healing. The website for loveyourbrain.org states that yoga

> [H]as the potential to transform the wellbeing of those living with brain injury by improving their ability to strengthen, and reconnect to, their mind and body. It can promote their acceptance of "what is" and help them recognize and appreciate their strengths, rather than focus on their perceived weaknesses.

This aligns with Dr. van der Kolk's writings and recommendations. He also has taught yoga at Kripalu Center for Yoga and Health in western Massachusetts (kripalu.org).

Shambhala Meditation Center of St. Johnsbury, Vermont, with which I've been involved, states: "Mindfulness/awareness meditation is the foundation of all that we do at the Shambhala Meditation Center. This ancient practice of self-discovery is rooted in the simple but revolutionary premise that every human being has the ability to cultivate the mind's inherent stability, clarity, and strength in order to be more awake and to develop the compassion and insight necessary to care for oneself and the world genuinely." Or as Jane Arthur of Karmê Chöling Shambhala Meditation Center in Vermont described it (as I include in this book) "courting oneself. When you take ten minutes a day to meditate, it's like checking in with a lover. Courtship is the ongoing nature of getting to know someone." And we never court ourselves, she said and I repeat. Truly getting to know yourself by appreciating your thoughts, nonjudgmentally—that can be achieved in meditation. "Mindfulness meditation encourages us to become more patient and compassionate with ourselves and to cultivate open-mindedness and gentle persistence," wrote Mark Williams and Danny Penman in *Mindfulness: An Eight-Week Plan for Finding Peace in a Frantic World*. Further, Sakyong Mipham writes in *Turning the Mind Into an Ally*, "The bewildered mind spends much of its time racing from distraction to distraction, from sound to sight to smell, from feeling to desire to disappointment. It's in a constant state of flirtation. On any given day, our consciousness is fragmented and scattered in all directions." This kind of inchoate existence may be tolerated by many who have accommodated white-knuckle navigation of mental chaos. However, peace, compassion, appreciation, and a settled mind are conducive to cognitive healing. Clinical evidence suggests that the human body plays an important role in this healing also.

EPILOGUE

BACK TO LIFE, AFTER THE FALL

I was meeting with my attending physician during a checkup a couple of months after my release from the rehab hospital when she asked me one of the standard doctor questions: Was I taking any medications at that time? I was no longer taking pain-relievers for my injured right arm and I was through (thankfully) with Colace to induce regularity following arm surgery. I'd had painful constipation for a week after my surgery, an apparent side effect of the surgical pain meds and anesthesia. When I told the doctor I was taking vitamins such as B-12, ginseng, and wild fish oil-Omega 3, it occurred to me to ask whether I should be taking something more. Anything more curative or potent for my cognitive recovery? Any neurological stimulator? Was there a brain panacea, a cognitive curative, I asked? The doctor asked me what I had in mind, so I said something like one of the behavioral meds we give to kids, nowadays—something like Adderall, but for brain function? Without missing a beat, she answered: No, they wouldn't prescribe anything like that, there was no special drug. She told me ginseng was probably okay. My answer was that I believed in it, that I had been taking it for years to improve my biorhythmic peaks. I had read, years before, that it provided mental energy and was a healthy stimulant. Maybe it would help with concentration and stamina, too, both of which were causing me struggles. Stamina seemed like a good idea to me, as my system would tire quickly as my brain fatigued. She said if I believed in it, she didn't see any reason not to keep taking it.

I began to increase my intake to copious amounts of *Panax ginseng*, or Asian ginseng, to about twenty-five hundred mg capsules a day. I also started ginkgo biloba, in addition to Omega 3 and B-12. Later, I added gotu kola, after I visited an herbal store and asked for "brain food." I was looking for something that friends from the Middle East in college referred to as *za'atar* and literally called it brain food. A soccer teammate from Saudi Arabia said they ate it when they studied, it was a mix of spices that they would spoon over foods or eat straight. I tried it once in college, and I remember it tasted like oregano. The herb store hadn't heard of this *za'atar* so instead I tried a gotu kola tea mixed with other herbs such as peppermint, rosemary, and Eleuthero root, which I could pack in a tea ball and steep in hot water.

I continued my clinical trial of vitamins and supplements for more than a year, at which point I thought to look into natural herbs used with Alzheimer's patients. My father has been prescribed donepezil HCI (brand name Aricept) for several years, as he is one of the more than five million Americans living with the condition. The drug appears to have arrested the progression of my father's Alzheimer's in the mild or moderate stage and he continues daily life, with the help of my mother. My thinking as a nonmedical layman was to possibly find an agent to help my own brain function, in the way donepezil HCI is thought to facilitate the production of acetylcholine, a neurotransmitter that promotes neurons firing together. An online search yielded three that I thought would be worth trying: Huperzine A (derived from Chinese moss), Vinpocetine (an extract from the lesser periwinkle plant), and DMAE or Deanol (dimethylaminoethanol bitartrate), which may form the neurotransmitter acetylcholine and aid in brain function. I took these for more than a year, on and off, and I can't swear to any definite brain-function improvement. Possibly, I gained some alertness—or maybe that was just moon phase or diet or biorhythms? Now that I've tried this clinical trial of vitamins and herbs, I simply don't want to stop taking them. I don't want to risk losing any abilities I've gained back during this time. (I also met with a holistic health practitioner and she recommended ashwagandha and multivitamins including vitamins D and B.) I haven't had doctors check the levels of dopamine or serotonin in my blood. I might be superstitious, or foolish to spend the money on these supplements. I feel this is something I can do, nutritionally, at least—and natural, not pharmaceutical.

I read an article in *The Challenge!*, the journal of the Brain Injury Association of America, that talked about drugs that might facilitate the growth of molecules in neurons that lead to synapses. The authors wrote, "We suspect that drugs that target CREB [one such molecule] could improve learning and memory after TBI by promoting the strengthening of synaptic connections." As I mentioned in the last chapter, perhaps we could achieve activation and growth of these molecules in our brains through meditation practice, instead of through meds? Our brains have plasticity—we can change brain functions if we work at them. It takes work and effort outside what modern life forces upon us, starting with a few minutes each day of peaceful abiding and courtship of oneself, as Jane Arthur so wonderfully put it. A simple focus on the breath is a way to start. This is a practice that's as old as time. Perhaps as the medical community often concludes: More studies are needed.

My medical recovery, in effect, ended when I was allowed to return to work in January 2013. The school's varsity basketball team was having a memorable year and the head coach, a former college coach, was driving and inspiring them to an undefeated season in Vermont Division I high school and the state-championship game, which the team lost in overtime. I felt a great sense of connection with the school at that time, and tremendous appreciation for the staff and faculty welcoming me back in January of that year. This buoyed me and provided personal support—and gave the all-important sense of normalcy the brain seeks out. We want to belong, we want to fit in, we want to contribute.

I can't overstate how important that sense of achieving normalcy is during recovery—inasmuch as a head-injured patient knows they function differently than they did before the injury, we want to be regarded as normal. You might never think about tying your shoelaces, it's a basic memory skill acquired at age three or four; however, I think differently now and think it's a pretty cool little skill to have acquired and mastered and leads to all manner of other hand-eye coordination and memory skills.

More than two years beyond the date of my injury, I still employ circumlocution as a conversational strategy. If I can't find the exact words for which I'm mentally searching to make a definite point, I keep talking until I complete the puzzle and express my thought. (Unless I lose my thought and have to say, "Where was I again?") I jokingly call it not having a governor; I probably sound verbose or chatty—or maybe nonsensical, sometimes. As I near the age of fifty, I figure this happens, with age, to everyone eventually. The phrase "senior moment" comes to mind. I'm mindful also that Alzheimer's is in my family, and that my father showed indications of it in his sixties, maybe even before that, though his family never knew. He probably did, but he's not saying now. Clearly, it's a condition in which the individual knows that he still knows—he is still *homo sapiens sapiens*—only he also knows he doesn't know in the same way he used to know.

I'm elated to say I have not slumped back into a compulsion for alcohol consumption. I no longer have an interior monologue so have no internal voice to quell. I no longer wrap myself up in the booze cocoon. In the past couple of years, I infrequently have had alcoholic drinks, and I know that when I do it's partly to appear normal. I don't crave the cognitive effects of alcohol. I don't like the effects. It actually scares me, a little. I respect the effects of booze, now. My sense is that this is what most normal drinkers feel—an inhibited respect for the effect. I continue to marvel at the (so to speak) lobotomized change in my behavior—I did have a frontal lobe injury to my brain, maybe there is some connection or correlation with a change of brain function in that I don't have the interior monologue as I did before, and therefore don't feel I need to seek any assistance with quieting my mind and my thoughts.

When I feel inner angst, I meditate. When I want to slow down, I meditate. When I need to give thanks for being alive, I meditate. I humbly appreciate and accept the beauty of life and all that's in it. "Behold the universe in the glory of God: and all that lives and moves on Earth" says the translation of the Isa Upanishad (which I began to study about two decades before my injury) that I've referenced repeatedly in this book. I face a paradox in my enjoyment of fishing and hunting—indeed, I edit a wingshooting magazine now, a sport that has the bittersweet result of the hunter killing a game bird. There is no catch-and-release wing shooting. That somber ending is tempered by the enjoyment of spending a day in the woods, watching my English pointer bird dog do what he loves—pursue the scent of game, instinctually—and I eat the meat of the dead birds, and use their plumage as fly-tying materials with which to make fishing flies. As the novelist and poet Jim Harrison said about hunting (and as a hunter himself), maybe we're just not as evolved as most people. I know it is the *being there* that I appreciate most, and the same is true when I feel the push of current on my legs while standing in a trout stream or wading through the tide in the ocean, with a fly rod in my right hand. To me, hunting and fishing are meditative pursuits. Anything that helps me—or forces me—to appreciate the beauty of life is meditative. I return once again to Rabindranath Tagore.

His poem "Brahma, Vishnu, Shiva" mentions "a new life exultant." I know that feeling, now.

My recovery continues and will through life, I'm quite sure. Maybe we're meant to acquire experience in the early stages of life, into our twenties, and then recover from that for the rest of our life, refining and recalibrating our internal equipment—our brain, our internal computer—till we finally are ready to let go. If the dreams created in amnesia by my amygdala were correct, I'll have an afterlife setting of quiet water and placid, tranquil happiness. I truly wish the same for you—celebrated now in life and lasting into the beyond.

I have to relate what's to me one more meaningful anecdote from my continuing life. One weekend in October 2014, as I was finishing a first draft of this manuscript, I was scheduled to attend a pheasant shoot and fly-fishing event at a private club in New Jersey. Organized by my friend the fine artist Peter Corbin (petercorbin.com), part of the proceeds would go to the American Museum of Fly Fishing in Vermont and Fort Ticonderoga in New York State. I left home on a rainy morning to begin the seven-hour drive south to New Jersey from Northern Vermont on Interstate 91. I was driving a rented 2014 Chevrolet Camaro and within an hour of my drive was pulled over for speeding; the Vermont state trooper told me he had clocked me at eighty-one miles an hour. I proceeded south, restrained now and with a heightened awareness of the horsepower of this vehicle. I set the cruise control at sixty-seven. The rain came down heavier on pace with the public radio weather report's warning of flooding in southern New Hampshire and parts of western Massachusetts. Rainwater was collecting on I-91, enough to make me take notice and stay toward the center lane, away from the highway shoulders. As I passed the Greenfield exit in Massachusetts, I was coming up quickly on a tractor-trailer truck in the right lane in front of me. Rather than test the antilock brakes, I eased into the left, passing lane and began to pass the truck.

When I opened my eyes, I was lying on my back being pushed into what appeared to be a small, white room. My arms felt restrained; when I turned my head to look at my right arm, it had a tube threaded into it. A man told me I had been in an accident, and he asked me simple questions, like the date and the time, and if I could think of which holiday was coming up. Halloween was the following weekend, I said. I asked what happened. Apparently, the car I was driving slammed into the guardrail after hydroplaning or fishtailing and I probably overcompensated with corrective steering and plunged the car under the truck's trailer. In doing so, I sheered off one of the truck's fuel tanks. My car was totaled, the ambulance driver, Jim, told me. I was very lucky, he said. I told him about my head injury and he asked me to sit tight and wait till we got to the hospital, to try to relax. I did. I could not remember the accident, any collision or impact, any perturbation in the forces of life, at all. One minute, I was passing the trailer; the next I was lying on my back on a stretcher in an ambulance with an IV in my arm. We pulled up to the emergency room in Springfield, Massachusetts, and I was wheeled inside for tests.

CT scans were the first order of business and I waited about an hour to be taken to the scanning room, my head clearing gradually but not triggering memory recall. I was groggy but didn't convulse or have any seizures. The traumatic event was missing from memory as if it never happened. I was cushioned through the impact—protected by airbags and the shoulder restraint seatbelt. I must have hit my head, hard enough to interrupt the limbic system or jolt the hippocampus. Could a whiplash effect have caused that? This was another episode of amnesia. How it was caused, I had no idea. I had no memory and I feared what the scan might reveal, still aware of seeing after the fact the scans taken at Dartmouth-Hitchcock Medical Center on August 14, 2012, showing bilateral intraparenchymal hemorrhages and intraventricular and subarachnoid blood and subdural fluid.

I had pain in my chest, where the seatbelt restrained me—or was that an injury to my internal organs or had I cracked the ribcage? I told the doctor about my chest pain, and he ordered body x-rays, in addition to the CT scans, but told me that if I broke or cracked ribs I would be much more than uncomfortable—I wouldn't be moving.

I waited, was given the tests, and waited more. I felt haunted by the missing memory, an eerie out-of-body sense that was still with me from the amnesia weeks I was told I had in 2012. I breathed deeply and meditated while lying on the gurney. A nurse told me I could make a phone call, so I called my wife, with whom I had spoken while I was on my back in the ambulance. My wife, a realtor, was home from her real-estate office that morning as our son didn't have school that day; once we spoke and she knew I was okay, she was practical in thinking about finding babysitting for our son if and when she had to come meet me in Massachusetts. She once again proved patient and compassionate and seemed to take this fateful episode in stride. (I know, baby—I will do all I can to keep this kind of moment out of our lives forevermore!) I was in a hospital about an hour from where she grew up, and she called my brother-in-law, who picked me up later at the hospital, after gathering my personal effects at a tow yard. That was after the doctors gave me the incredibly good news that my CT scan was normal. The findings read: "Brain: No parenchymal hemor-rhage, midline shift or mass effect. Ventricles, cisterns, and sulci are normal. Gray-white matter differentiation is well preserved." All was normal. So were the body x-rays. I was discharged and my brother-in-law took me to his and my sister-in-law's house. As my wife said in a deadpan way, I had dodged a bullet.

Knowing how fragile the head and brain can be—well-shielded by the skull, but that can change in an instant—I can clinically say about this car wreck: I was incredibly lucky. On August 14, 2012, the findings of a CT scan indicated very different outcomes: "There are multiple, bifrontal intraparenchymal hemorrhages, the largest in the left frontal lobe measuring 3.2 x 2.8 cm. There is likely subdural blood along the falx, subarachnoid blood is present within the right tempo-ral lobe, and there is intraventricular blood in the left temporal horn. Minimal subdural fluid/blood overlying the right convexity note. A small focus of hemorrhage is seen within the left basal ganglia, as well as within the left lateral ventricle. . . There is no skull facture."

But the brain is protected, still. I had walked away from the car crash—and eventually I had resumed life after my plummet from the tree or ladder. And life has never been more meaningful or fulfilling.

I'm a habitual tea drinker these days, warming my esophageal tract, soothing my stomach, and satisfying the need to relax and focus with "the cup that cheers but doesn't" as Sean O'Casey called tea in his masterwork *Juno and the Paycock*. What serendipity tonight when I poured the hot water over a bag of ginger tea and noticed an aphorism attached to the tea bag, as is the custom of Yogi brand teas—the message read: "The purpose of life is to enjoy every moment."

That stopped me cold in my tracks. I thought about it and had a shallow laugh. This is a statement of existence for me now, a mission statement of sorts. And inasmuch as I've always had a tropism toward the beauty of life, I can't say I always valued the beauty of being alive or lived that way. I don't know why. Sunsets, music, laughter, calm water, flowing rivers, a gentle breeze, the still of the night— I value and love these. I love family; I love my son and my wife. I love the simplicity of existence. I've puzzled over why we make life so complicated and hard—even as I did just that for many years. It seemed the harder and more complicated I made life, the greater the challenge living was, and I relished that challenge. I no longer accept that.

I marvel at my memories of fly fishing for Atlantic salmon in the Cathedral Pool on the River Moy in the northwestern Irish town of Ballina, County Mayo, the exulted and ecstatic feeling I had with each flip of my Spey rod amid the rushing swell of river music echoing off the retaining wall along the river's edge; or the infinite joy I experienced on March 13–14, 2008, in the birthing pool with Robin when our son was born in Maine. I still have these memories, my brain preserved them—I can recall them.

How do I think differently since my brain trauma? My thinking has expanded, my consciousness has opened up.

I feel living simply is a reward. Simply living is, too.

I know we have to care for those we love, letting them know how we feel. Love is powerful, and just saying or thinking the word releases emotions. Talk about love, freely. It's powerful and empowering. Never mind trying to be right, or trying always to win. In my life so far, I squandered years with calculations and exertions on these two efforts, overpowered by ego.

Be fair, respectful and friendly, be open and accessible. Share. Give and don't hesitate to receive. Humility, kindness, and understanding are three of the most potent values in life. And love. I fell, I struck my head, I recovered, and now I appreciate these elements of life more than ever, greatly and deeply. To you, I truly wish, in the words of the Isa Upanishad: Find joy in the Eternal. To my loved ones, to my son and my wife—I love you.

BRAIN INJURY ORGANIZATIONS

Acoustic Neuroma Association
600 Peachtree Parkway
Suite 108
Cumming, GA 30041
info@anausa.org
http://www.anausa.org
Tel: (770) 205-8211/ (877) 200-8211
Fax: (770) 205-0239/ (877) 202-0239

Brain Injury Association of America, Inc.
1608 Spring Hill Road
Suite 110
Vienna, VA 22182
braininjuryinfo@biausa.org
http://www.biausa.org
Tel: (703) 761-0750/ (800) 444-6443
Fax: (703) 761-0755

Brain Trauma Foundation
1 Broadway
6th Floor
New York, NY 10004
education@braintrauma.org
www.braintrauma.org
Tel: (212) 772-0608
Fax: (212) 772-0375

Family Caregiver Alliance/National Center on Caregiving
785 Market St.
Suite 750
San Francisco, CA 94103
info@caregiver.org
www.caregiver.org
Tel: (415) 434-3388/ (800) 445-8106
Fax: (415) 431-3508

National Rehabilitation Information Center (NARIC)
8201 Corporate Drive
Suite 500
Landover, MD 20785
naricinfo@heitechservices.com
www.naric.com
Tel: (301) 459-5900/ (301) 459-5981
TTY: (800) 364-2742
Fax: (301) 562-2401

National Stroke Association
9707 East Easter Lane
Suite B
Centennial, CO 80112
info@stroke.org
www.stroke.org

Tel: (303) 649-9299/ (800) 787-6537
Fax: (303) 649-1328

National Institute on Disability and Rehabilitation Research (NIDRR)
U.S. Department of Education Office of Special Education and Rehabilitative Services
400 Maryland Ave., S.W.
Washington, DC 20202-7100
www.ed.gov/about/offices/list/osers/nidrr
Tel: (202) 245-7460/ (202) 245-7316

RESOURCES

Rehabilitation and Recovery

I personally found that hard work, dedication to achievement, and perseverance were key factors in my recovery from brain injury, once I regained consciousness and could create and retain memories again, as well as recall previous memories. I'm quite sure I'll never get back any detail from that nearly month of amnesia I had in August and a couple of days in September 2012; but as the doctors told me, not a whole lot happened anyway, only boring medical stuff—and I did hold on to the powerful escapist dreams I had during that period.

I was driven to do the best I could at the simple tasks with which I began recovery, and kept that personal commitment along the way as the tasks became more difficult—which led to a return to at least a version of everyday life after about five months. I continued to improve, if not every day, certainly month by month. As I write this, I feel stronger than ever; by the end of this week, I'll probably be incrementally better, unless I have a lapse in cognitive ability, which is normal to human life. We all have ups and downs, highs and lows—but one of the most important aspects following a brain injury is maintaining our determination to improve.

From a medical point of view, in *Communicating Prognosis (Core Principles of Acute Neurology)*, Dr. Eelco F. M. Wijdicks of the Mayo Clinic, writes:

> Every practitioner in this field knows that patients with large contusions, early brain edema, and initial poor neurological condition may still make a substantial improvement in a matter of months after TBI. The doctor does advocate for evaluation of the type of injury lending some determination of the course and duration of treatment.

With that fixed in mind, family members of brain-injury patients or the patients themselves will benefit from knowing as much as possible about the injury and brain function. I recommend the following:

Traumatic Brain Injury Assistance Books

Chicken Soup for the Soul series
Recovering from Traumatic Brain Injuries: 101 Stories of Hope, Healing, and Hard Work
Amy Newmark and Dr. Carolyn Roy-Bornstein
Chicken Soup for the Soul Publishing
P.O. Box 700
Cos Cob, CT 06807

Communicating Prognosis (Core Principles of Acute Neurology)
Eelco F. M. Wijdicks, M.D., Ph.D., FNCS, FANA
Professor of Neurology, Mayo Clinic College of Medicine
Chair, Division of Critical Care Neurology
Consultant, Neurosciences Intensive Care Unit Saint Marys Hospital, Mayo Clinic, Rochester, Minnesota
Oxford University Press
198 Madison Avenue, New York, NY 10016

Handling Difficult Situations (Core Principles of Acute Neurology)
Eelco F. M. Wijdicks, M.D., Ph.D., FNCS, FANA
Professor of Neurology, Mayo Clinic College of Medicine
Chair, Division of Critical Care Neurology
Consultant, Neurosciences Intensive Care Unit Saint Marys Hospital,
Mayo Clinic, Rochester, Minnesota
Oxford University Press
198 Madison Avenue, New York, NY 10016

Providing Acute Care (Core Principles of Acute Neurology)
By Eelco F. M. Wijdicks, M.D., Ph.D., FNCS, FANA
Professor of Neurology, Mayo Clinic College of Medicine
Chair, Division of Critical Care Neurology Consultant, Neurosciences
Intensive Care Unit Saint Marys Hospital, Mayo Clinic, Rochester,
Minnesota
Oxford University Press, 198 Madison Avenue, New York, NY 10016

Head Cases: Stories of Brain Injury and Its Aftermath
Michael Paul Mason
Farrar, Straus and Giroux
18 West 18th Street, New York, NY 10011

Cognition, Cognitive Research, and Brain Function Information

The Brain That Changes Itself: Stories of Personal Triumph from the Frontiers of Brain Science
Norman Doidge, M.D.
Penguin Books
375 Hudson Street, New York, NY 10014

A Calm Brain: Unlocking Your Natural Relaxation System
Gayatri Devi, M.D.
Dutton, a member of the Penguin Group
375 Hudson Street, New York, NY 10014

In an Instant: A Family's Journey of Love and Healing
Lee and Bob Woodruff
Random House Publishing Group
1745 Broadway, New York, NY 10019

In Search of Memory: The Emergence of a New Science of Mind
Eric R. Kandel
W.W. Norton & Company
500 Fifth Avenue, New York, NY 10110

My Stroke of Insight: A Brain Scientist's Personal Journey
Jill Bolte Taylor, Ph.D.
Viking Press, a member of Penguin Group
375 Hudson Street, New York, NY 10014

Rewire Your Brain: Think Your Way to a Better Life
John B. Arden, Ph.D.
John Wiley & Sons, Inc.
111 River Street, Hoboken, NJ 07030

The Mind & The Brain: Neuroplasticity and the Power of Mental Force
Jeffrey M. Schwartz and Sharon Begley
HarperCollins Publishers
10 East 53rd Street, New York, NY 10022

Synaptic Self: How Our Brains Become Who We Are
Joseph LeDoux
Penguin Group
375 Hudson Street, New York, NY 10014

Training the Brain: Cultivating Emotional Skills (part of the *Wired to Connect: Dialogues on Social Intelligence* series)
Daniel Goleman with Richard Davidson
More Than Sound LLC
221 Pine Street
Suite 408
Florence, MA 01062

The Tell-Tale Brain: A Neuroscientist's Quest for What Makes Us Human
V.S. Ramachandran
W.W. Norton & Company, Inc.
500 Fifth Avenue, New York, NY 10110

Meditation and Emotional Recovery

An Unquiet Mind: A Memoir of Moods and Madness
Kay Redfield Jamison
Picador, a member of the Macmillian Group
175 Fifth Avenue New York, NY 10010

The Enlightened Mind: An Anthology of Sacred Prose
Edited by Stephen Mitchell
HarperCollins Publishers
10 East 53rd Street, New York, NY 10022

The Mind's Own Physician: A Scientific Dialogue with the Dalai Lama on the Healing Power of Meditation
Edited by Jon Kabat-Zinn, PhD, and Richard J. Davidson, PhD, with Zara Houshmand
Mind and Life Institute,
New Harbinger Publications
5674 Shattuck Avenue, Oakland, CA 94609

The Organized Mind: Thinking Straight in the Age of Information Overload
Daniel Levitin
Dutton, Penguin Group
375 Hudson Street
New York, NY 10014

The Shambhala Principle: Discovering Humanity's Hidden Treasure
Sakyong Mipham
Harmony Books, Crown Publishing Group
1745 Broadway
New York, NY 10019

Living Beautifully with Uncertainty and Change
Pema Chodron
Shambhala Publications
Horticultural Hall
300 Massachusetts Avenue, Boston, MA 02115

Mindfulness: An Eight-Week Plan for Finding Peace in a Frantic World
Mark Williams and Danny Penman
Rodale, Inc.
733 Third Avenue, New York, NY 10017

Turning the Mind Into an Ally
Sakyong Mipham
Riverhead Books, a member of the Penguin Group
375 Hudson Street, New York, NY 10014

General Reading

A Lifetime of Vermont People
Peter Miller
Silver Print Press
20 Crossroad, Waterbury, VT 05676
www.silverprintpress.com

Selected Poems
Rabindranath Tagore
Penguin Books USA
375 Hudson Street, New York, NY 10014

The Spare Room
Jenny Land
Voyage, Brigantine Media
211 North Avenue, St. Johnsbury, VT 05819
www.brigantinemedia.com

The Way Back
Wyn Cooper
White Pine Press
P.O. Box 236, Buffalo, NY 14201
www.whitepine.org

The Upanishads
Juan Mascaro
Penguin Books USA
375 Hudson Street, New York, NY 10014